The Theory of

Social

Disruption

The Theory of
Social
Disruption

COL. Damon T. Arnold, M.D., M.P.H.

authorHOUSE®

AuthorHouse™
1663 Liberty Drive
Bloomington, IN 47403
www.authorhouse.com
Phone: 1-800-839-8640

Published by AuthorHouse   11/14/2012

ISBN: 978-1-4772-5943-6 (sc)
ISBN: 978-1-4772-5945-0 (hc)
ISBN: 978-1-4772-5944-3 (e)

Library of Congress Control Number: 2012914740

Table of Contents

To every sentient being

OZYMANDIAS

I met a traveler from an antique land
Who said: Two vast and trunkless legs of stone
Stand in the desert. Near them, on the sand,
Half sunk, a shattered visage lies, whose frown
And wrinkled lip, and sneer of cold command
Tell that its sculptor well those passions read
Which yet survive, stamped on the lifeless things,
The hand that mocked them and the heart that fed.
And on the pedestal these words appear:
"My name is Ozymandias, king of kings:
Look on my works, ye Mighty, and despair!"
Nothing beside remains. Round the decay
Of that colossal wreck, boundless and bare
The lone and level sands stretch far away.

Percy Bysshe Shelly (1792–1822)

Foreword

This book encompasses a wide array of topics that provide keen insights into how to implement community-based interventions. Several theoretical models are presented that help the readers to organize their thoughts and perceptions about the communities they are interacting with. The book also does an excellent job of explaining and blending the concepts of Eastern and Western scientific thought. These models create a framework for the further elucidation, study, and exploration of community engagement operational issues. It moves in a direction that sets the stage for addressing community-based infrastructure problems on both the emergent as well as the non-emergent basis with practical solutions.

The concepts contained within this book provide an approach to address some of the most urgent social conditions facing American citizens today. Further, it outlines some key principles and concepts, which Col. Damon T. Arnold notes were developed by federal agencies involved in homeland protection and security initiatives. Ample references are provided for the readers to broaden their knowledge base and to participate in formal online training. This book also serves as a reference document for those involved in both everyday and emergent social circumstances calling for orchestrating response activities.

Through the provision of anecdotal stories, Arnold provides rare glimpses into real-life considerations that serve as a basis for future policy developments and intervention approaches. The author also welcomes challenges to his theoretical underpinnings and practical applications. He notes that all theories are fluid in nature and should ultimately be responsive to the actual needs attended to within a community setting.

COL. Damon T. Arnold, M.D., M.P.H.

Arnold notes that it is essential for responders to use best practice models. He then also mentions that the responder must also keep in mind that situational awareness provides essential guidance for responses that lead to effective outcomes. The ability for systems to maintain an innate degree of flexibility is also stressed as being essential for ensuring the success of operationally efficient and effective interventions.

Further, Arnold notes that every citizen has a responsibility to extinguish the flames of social injustice and to support and strengthen our nation. It is clearly stated that the positive values and morals, as well as American ingenuity and innovation, underlie the future ascendancy of our great nation.

Russel L. Honore
Lieutenant General
US Army (Ret.)

Acknowledgments

I would like to dedicate this book to several people. First and foremost, I dedicate it to my parents, Dorothy Sinclair Arnold and Charles William Arnold. They were both hard working and talented people who survived the civil rights struggles to gain recognition as truly exceptional American citizens.

My father became a sheet-metal worker after returning from the WWII as a combat soldier and drill instructor in the US Army. Despite this, he wore the stigma in America of being inferior because of his skin color. This deeply affected his choices in life and even where he was physically allowed to go. He was a war hero who was treated like an outcast as the result of a deranged social ideology, akin to that of the Nazi SS, which he fought against overseas. He lived as a dedicated American citizen, despite the hatred being hurled his way by many of the "good citizens" he protected.

My mother was a gifted social worker who exemplified what I consider to be the highest form of human development possible. She was not only a genius but also adept at combining her passion with compassion. This resulted in the creation of miracles in the lives of multitudes of people of all races, ethnicities, and creeds, whom she encountered. She did this until her death at 91 years of age.

I remember my mother introducing me when I was very young to people that she rented rooms to in our four-story brownstone home in Brooklyn, New York. She told me they were my relatives, whom I needed to deeply respect and that she was renting rooms to them. While a student in the sixth grade, I saw her struggling with paying the bills one day. She was worried that we were going to lose our home. I then asked her why she charged them so little for rent. I realized that she charged them barely 10 percent of what was being charged for rooms of the same type in the area. She retorted angrily to me, "Shut your mouth and keep quiet!"

Later I discovered that these were families in trouble. As a consummate social worker, she was stabilizing these families so that they could recover from lost jobs or even to restore to them a will to live. These 'relatives' would then regain their strength, keep their relationships together, and move back into life. She prayed every day for love, tolerance, and peace to enter the world. No greater legacy or accomplishment can a human being leave on the face of the earth than this.

If there is any rival in such a pursuit it would be my wife, Sharon Johnson-Arnold, who has a heart of gold. She has seen me through my demanding work schedules as well as my multiple deployments to global regions and war zones during my military career. She is not only the wind beneath my wings but also the embodiment of the very spirit the world so desperately needs today. She is a consummate professional and a compassionate spirit to all.

Truly inspirational in my life were my aunts and uncles, Theodore and George Sinclair, Joan and Jack Jackson, and Avis and June Mulveny. Also I acknowledge my cousins Barbara, Kathy, and Wesley Jackson, who have provided wisdom and guidance that deeply enriched my earthly existence.

I would also like to thank my brother and sister, David and Verona. In addition, I am truly blessed to have and am deeply proud of my nephews, Christopher, Jason, Alex, Tommy, and Tyler as well as my nieces, Leah, Nicole, Mya, and Sandhya. My brothers—and sisters-in-law, Thomas and Lorraine Lynch and Rodney and Stephanie Gaston, and my mother-in-law, Pearline Haywood, have enriched my life, and I am very proud of all their accomplishments. Baby Evan Bowers, who currently seems to be hooked on dinosaurs, has added great joy to the entire family.

I would like to acknowledge the tremendous contributions made by the men and women of all branches of the Armed Forces and well as the Center for Homeland Defense and Security in Monterey, CA. These individuals are as much a part of my family as my own flesh and blood relatives.

Without mentors, colleagues, and friends, we would be a mere pile of celestial dust. I would like to especially thank Dr. Cheryl and Dr. Eric Whitaker, Quin and Victor Golden, Dr. Carl Bell, Rev. Janette Wilson, JD, Joseph Harrington, Rory Slater, Mildred Hunter, Dr. Paul Jarris, Commissioner Michelle Saddler, Col. Eugene Blackwell, Floretta Strong-Pulley, Dr. Teifu Shen, and Dr. Ma for their support, wisdom, and phenomenal friendships. Dr. Eric Witaker and Quin Golden in particular have been consummate, visionary professionals who have saved countless lives and prevented the occurrence of pain, suffering, and death in the lives of millions of citizens.

I admire and commend the Reverend Jesse L. Jackson Sr. and his family for endless contributions to the civil and human rights struggles and accomplishments for which we all are beneficiaries. Congressman Bobby Rush and Louanner Peters have been beacons and effective leaders in the battles against inequity for our citizens. There are also pioneers for justice and role models of perfection embodied in such icons as Congressman Daniel ("Danny") and his wife Vera Davis. Without these heroes we all would be mere shadows of what we have been enabled by their efforts to become.

It is rare to have such colleagues and supportive friends as I do with doctors such as Judy and Lester Munson, Michael Seng, Pieku Tu, Cheryl Lin, and Chih-Liang Yaung. Dr. Munson and Dr. Seng have contributed greatly to the fields of international and constitutional law and emergency preparedness efforts on a global scale. Dr. Tu and Dr. Lin, through their program at Duke University, have heralded the creation of international cooperation and understanding. Dr. Yaung, who previously directed the Taiwan national public health system, is visionary, dedicated, passionate, and brilliant. His legacy will be one of presenting a global view of how to build and put into operation an outstanding and effective information technology-based public health system.

COL. Damon T. Arnold, M.D., M.P.H.

I would also like to acknowledge Jack Lynch, Charisse Witherspoon, and Ellen Rozelle-Turner for their tremendous support and friendship. I would be lost without colleagues such as doctors Elton Tinsley, Paul Brandt-Rauf, Georges Benjamin, Terry Mason, and Monique and Stephen Martin as well as attorneys Charles Nesbitt and George Jackson who provide wisdom, friendship, and phenomenal support. They are all consummate professionals and have made enormous contributions to the health of our nation's citizens.

Finally, I would like to thank Lt. Gen. Russel Honore, who wrote the foreword for this book. He is the "John Wayne dude" that saved the day during Hurricane Katrina's wrath. He not only made a tremendous impact in mitigating pain and suffering and saving countless lives during that disaster but protected our nation throughout a brilliant military career. He is truly an American hero, role model, and national icon we should all make an attempt to emulate. Make sure to go online and learn about this remarkable soldier, citizen, and, indeed, national treasure known as Lt. Gen. Russel Honore.

I am truly grateful that each of the individuals noted above has chosen to make invaluable contributions to humanity as well as to my personal experiences. Without their presence in my life, I would be lost and decidedly less than I am—that is, if I would have survived at all without their presence.

Preface

This book encompasses the journey of exploration I have been involved in over several decades. I have presented several concepts, many of which I have created in an attempt to order the complexities encountered along the way. They serve as a framework for further study and exploration of the world that surrounds us as well as our inner selves.

It must be kept in mind that no theory withstands the scrutiny of time as more information unfolds about any identified issues. As we discover new information, it redefines the very elements that serve as the basis for our earlier explanatory constructs. The question becomes whether validation is just a stone's throw away from what we recognize as truth. Is the very process of validation too innately strained by our perceptions of what we think reality is to be truly a valid process? Reaching the perfection of an ability to causally ascribe to an intervention strategy a particular outcome would be unobtainable. This stride toward perfection merely is an ongoing process that borders upon and is guided by the realm of philosophical thought and the practical applications of the art of science.

Yet, at various junctures along the way, one is able to feel a certain level of satisfaction and reward. This sense emerges from the fruition of successful, goal-orientated accomplishments. To that end, hopefully the reader finds the information contained in this book useful. I have attempted to provide concepts related to self-development, Eastern-Western scientific thought, and a deeper understanding of community-based settings. In addition, I have provided emergency-response concepts and some potential intervention model platforms. This information is essential for anyone working to improve the social conditions of the citizens within our country.

COL. Damon T. Arnold, M.D., M.P.H.

While serving in military medicine practice, I have had the opportunity to have missions in Central America, South America, Africa, Europe, the Middle East, and Asia. I have interwoven some of these experiences in this book to add an element of realism to the concepts I have attempted to describe. Integrate the concepts in this book with knowledge you currently possess. And voraciously challenge the concepts, as this is the only way to truly make progress.

All too often students are instructed not to think, but rather to memorize facts and to subsequently regurgitate them on paper. There is little thought, creativity, or imagination involved, if any, in such a process. Further, the lack of a true comprehension of the presented materials leads to poor communication and a deadened sense of inquiry on the part of the student.

Conventional thought and wisdom undeniably have their merits and strong points. However, many of the views I have presented are meant to foster the development of independent thought and the ability to think unfettered by ritualistic, dogmatic viewpoints. Note also that it is just as important to redefine the view of one's true self as it is to redefine concepts of one's encounters.

I would also be remiss not to mention what I feel to be a fundamental requirement for those concerned with improving society in our nation as it currently exists. Today, our constitutional crucible is challenged as we attempt to extinguish the flames of social injustice that deteriorate our values, morals, and integrity.

Throughout history, these flames have engendered and perpetuated the death spirals of disparity based upon ethnicity, race, gender, age, economic class, sexual orientation, ideologies, and religious belief systems. Despite this, our ancestors have broken some of these chains of violence, hatred, and abuse to varying degrees. Indeed, many have lost their lives in defense of this morally based action, so that we may even exist at all.

Many champions have striven to ignite the torch of social justice, affording us tremendous amounts of success and historical resiliency in combating social injustice. This has occurred on a global scale. We should move forward using these instruments our ancestors have crafted for us.

There is a continuing and urgent need to illuminate and focus upon unethical and immoral social and policy practices that foster inequities and, in so doing, extinguish them. Such primitive practices reflect a state of moral bankruptcy and mental insanity on the parts of those who would practice them. Truly, their amassed legacy is an attempt to demoralize the very principles of trust, honesty, morality, and good will for all people. As true interventionists, we must stand in full opposition to such practices. In addition, the lack of education and the cultural brainwashing engendered by such practices provide fertile soil for the sowing of the seeds of discontent, rage, violence, and anger.

These practices initially place kinks in the armor of the integrity of individual and collective community members. Finally, the consequences from such practices coil around the very souls of those contained within disparately impacted communities, yielding disastrous results. This leads to the social marginalization of targeted subgroups, which then further kindles social disruption and thereby ensures the materialization and perpetuation of the death spirals of disparity. In fact, Stage IV physical and mental illness and disease are inextricably linked to Stage IV social disruption within our communities.

All too often, this has resulted in the encasement within concrete prison walls of the very hearts and souls of our children globally. Such disruption is the subject of this book. Often this originates in the framework of an underlying institutionalized inequity that is pervasive and echoes within our communities. Always remember that ignorance, unconscious bias, stereotyping, and discrimination are the lynchpins of hatred-filled ideologies.

In fact, these destructive ideologies threaten and suppress the right to be heard, the will to be happy, and the very right to be free from physical and mental illness and disease. Essentially, these ideologies threaten the existence of the very things humans hold to be precious—indeed, priceless. Such ideologies are fundamentally unconstitutional and diametrically opposed to the principles underlying good mental, emotional, and physical health.

However, some of our ancestors did not sink within the quicksand of this immorality imparted by hatred-filled demagogues. Rather, they attempted to replace the tombstones of social injustice and despair. They did this by paving the pathways for social justice and the construction of the monuments of love, respect, and dignity within our communities. For they understood that within such a realm, artistic beauty, grace, peace, and hope could flourish for all. In times of war and as public servants for the protection of our heritage as human beings, they did not hesitate to perform their duties with personal sacrifice, even unto death. They came to the defense of those who were most vulnerable and wrongfully persecuted.

Remember that, within this very country, the constant marching to the cemetery of peoples' dignity, hopes, and dreams was reversed by a drum major for justice. Dr. Martin Luther King Jr. used his faith in both a higher power and in humanity as well as an operational philosophy of nonviolence as his tools. His rallying cry for a national collective consciousness, based on ethical principles and moral values, made us see that "injustice anywhere is a threat to justice everywhere." His global impact for the betterment of all humanity was self-evident. Likewise, it is everyone's ethical and moral imperative to eradicate the roots of inequity and its consequential social injustices and disparate impacts. This is especially true for those that live as citizens within these communities or practice public health and the healing arts.

One must continue to march forward with an indomitable spirit. This is especially true when one attempts to repair and heal the societal pathways and constructs so important to the ultimate happiness, health, and very survival of all citizens. One must also strive to ensure the restoration of the vestments of respect, security, justice, and liberty for all human beings on a global scale. Many of these individuals have been the victims of externally imposed, self-destructive ideologies and misfortunes.

One must be mindful to protect and nurture the developing minds of all his or her young on a global scale. There must be installed within them a sense of honor, humility, respect, and compassion for all others they meet. They must also be taught to respect both the natural and health-oriented, man-made environments that surround them.

This frame of reference must be borne in mind as future generations fulfill their duties to our society as a global whole. To do less would be tantamount to a molestation of the efforts and prophetic voices of those who carried the torches of social justice and good will throughout history.

Remember that unbridled passion can also be used for an evil purpose. Therefore, passion must always be mixed with compassion when creating policies and intervention plans. This is extremely important, as their very application will impact individuals who are victims of unfortunate circumstances. This is particularly true when an outside group reaches into a community in an attempt to respond to its needs. It is the fusion of passion, compassion, and effective community engagements, that gives rise to the actions that result in effective community healing interventions.

Although we are a world of multiple ancient origins and descents, together every person must set ablaze and maintain the torch of social justice for all sentient beings. Each person must recall our ultimate commonality. Never underestimate one's dedication and resolve to accomplish this very thing.

Society as a whole must secure the rallying points for peaceful public discourse and debate. Members of society must not be afraid to speak up against human rights and justice violations on a local as well as a global scale. The global society must express a lack of tolerance for hate-based ideologies anywhere on Earth. This also requires unwavering support for the elimination of inequities and disparities wherever they occur.

The global society must stand together at the helm in facing our ethical and spiritual destiny. Each person must reignite his or her personal sense of humanity by supporting all human beings globally. This is especially true for those who may be disparately impacted or have special needs. Move forward with passion, but never forget the essential ingredient of compassion for others and oneself.

One must promote and support global unity, as this is the only way for the world to truly heal. Remember that without this, Earth as a planet might not survive at all. In fact, without this, all our other tools are ineffective and, quite frankly, worthless. This is because you will have failed to recognize the human spirit within those you have touched or have attempted to touch.

With this is mind, I wish you a healthy, spiritually uplifting, and miraculous journey throughout your lifetime.

Introduction

The Theory of Social Disruption

Americans, who spring from multiple origins, races, and ethnicities, all face one common challenge—that is, the vast majority of illnesses, diseases, and injuries people face within our nation are often the result of self-inflicted individual and collective behaviors.

Together Americans must overcome this death spiral by resetting the behavioral compass of this nation to create a healthier cultural paradigm. For this to occur, the focus must be on the attainment of the best possible health outcome for society as a whole. This nation can achieve optimum health outcomes only by renewing the collective commitment to minimize morbidity (pain and suffering) and premature mortality (early, preventable deaths). Furthermore, this self-inflicted form of social disruption not only results in avoidable pain, suffering, and premature deaths, but in the erosion of our communities and the nation as a whole. It burdens medical and social service systems, decreases property values, and reduces productivity. It negatively impacts the citizens' health and the nation's fiscal stability.

In recent decades, there has been an alarming increase in both the prevalence and the associated chronic disease burden of obesity in the United States. This calls into question the very future stability and existence of our nation. The decisions made now will define the direction the health of future generations will take. Americans can no longer ignore or fiscally afford the devastating personal and social consequences of self-inflicted diseases and preventable injuries.

COL. Damon T. Arnold, M.D., M.P.H.

As we face this societal problem, each individual is personally responsibility to assist in this process. Yet as Americans establish healing pathways and travel toward a common destiny, it is also crucial to reignite the torch of social justice. Blindness and indifference to the pain and suffering of others will lead people further astray into social disruption and despair as a societal collective. This is especially true when confronting the needs of disparately impacted subpopulations.

Public health officials and academic institutions are charged with creating policies to support community programs designed to eliminate disease on a population-based level. However, these policies often end up as useless collections of paper on the shelves without any apparent connection to a truly "operationalized" intervention strategy. They are most often never put into action; they are merely data-driven historical documentations of the results of watchful inaction. However, not all caves are without candles. I sincerely hope that a concerted effort is made by academia to learn how to strike the match that allows the candle of useful and effective community engagement to be lit.

Academic documents must be translated into actionable steps, and community engagement is essential for any plan to succeed. A lack of engagement has actually ruined many community intervention plans. The development of a strong degree of community engagement is critical to efforts directed at the restoration or establishment of community stability and resiliency.

Indeed, much of what is done in public health is focused on the provision of Stage IV treatment. However, little attention is paid to the combined effects of the various components of a disrupted community environment. These disruptive factors clearly have direct impacts on illness, disease, and injury outcomes. This is explained in more detail in *Chapter 7—The Missing Line for Social Disruption.*

This book launches a new operations platform for the implementation of public health intervention strategies that require the integration of several conceptual viewpoints. These viewpoints are discussed in detail and then simplified so we can consider their respective roles. This conceptual model considers community member perspectives derived from direct engagement and "buy-in" for it to succeed. Community member perspectives are of paramount importance. Community engagement and realistically constructed intervention tools are required in order to effectively address community-based health problems. It is equally important to put these tools into use.

Any level of social disruption that has the potential for producing inordinate pain and suffering or a premature death is a potential target for intervention. This includes disruptions such as endemic illnesses, diseases, and injuries, whether of man-made or natural origin. This challenges the basis for the various roles that Critical Infrastructure and Key Resource (CIKR) sectors play. It extends from the basic necessities of life to established economic and political systems.

Agents that lead to morbidity and premature mortality arise within a continuous "energy-matter" spectrum. I crafted this viewpoint to explain the natural environment that surrounds us. This concept is explained in great detail in *Chapter 5—The Eastern-Western Bridge* and *Chapter 6—The Environmental Link to Your Health*. These agents arise within the context of a community environment that has a vacillating and relative degree of social order. The underlying degree of social order can strongly modify the effects of the various agents encountered. This can be either in a positive or a negative direction with respect to community member health outcomes subsequently observed.

The degree of social order is closely aligned with and arises from the CIKR sectors that surround us all. It also involves the factors that are known to be the social determinants of health, which are related to the relative risk prediction for an unhealthy outcome.

The relative degree of social order directly impacts community members. When this occurs in disparate ways, the affected subgroups can be placed into categories. These categories represent the social determinants of health. They are determinative of the morbidity and premature mortalities experienced within a community, based upon a common feature of those affected by exposure to one or more environmental agents.

If the sun is shining and one is especially prone to the development of skin cancer, one may elect to apply a sun-blocking lotion. However, if one is in an area where the business community infrastructure that does not provide for the acquisition of sunscreen products, one will be at higher risk for the development of skin cancer. The sunlight is the agent causing the skin cancer, but the infrastructure is not ordered in a way that protects those especially at risk for skin cancer by providing the sun-blocking lotion.

At first glance, a particular source of disruption may be viewed as having a limited and isolated impact. For example, the current trend regarding obesity in our nation is to focus upon the physical consequences impacting the afflicted individuals themselves. We simply look at it as the morbidity and premature mortality that occurs within an individual or group of people. However, obesity is not only a threat to the individual afflicted but also to the local community and the nation as a whole.

At a nationally televised conference in the spring of 2009 in Washington, DC, I noted that obesity threatened our nation at both the national and the domestic security levels. Secretaries Sebelius, Napolitano, and Duncan, as well as many federal and health-related officials, were present. I noted that obesity-related conditions disqualify recruited individuals at the induction physicals required for potential active and reserve military and National Guard service. They also exclude potential candidates who fail to meet physical requirements for service in domestic fire, police, emergency responder, and labor pools. Therefore, obesity is a direct national and domestic security threat. Many of the morbidities stemming from the occurrence of obesity, place an alarming burden on our national health care and financial systems. Obesity also places an inordinate burden on the family members of afflicted individuals.

Consider the prospect of an obese, single parent suffering a heart attack, resulting in hospitalization or even death. Children may go unattended and even be unaware of what has happened to their parent. The absence of the afflicted caregiver places these children at higher risk for exposure to violence. This is especially true within an impoverished and disordered inner-city environment. In this scenario, societal, geopolitical, and personal adjustment factors may have combined to increase the risk for the development of obesity. This set the stage for the development of heart disease. In turn this led to a crisis situation in which the safety of children was compromised. Therefore, the occurrence of the poor health consequences related to obesity in a parent may cause at-risk children to become vulnerable to violence. The point I wish to make is that these seemingly unrelated occurrences are actually interdependent and highly interrelated.

It then becomes obvious that, to address both national and domestic security concerns resulting from obesity, we must address this public health issue with a multidisciplinary approach. Obesity itself is a man-made disaster with implications on a global scale. The potential social consequences of obesity, based upon interactions with other societal factors, require further delineation. Obesity also has tremendous implications for the global economy.

In an inner-city environment, obesity arises within the context of 'food deserts,' which are blighted community settings where healthy food is unavailable. Actually, there is often easy access to dangerous food products. There is little practical difference between the effects of poisons or chemical warfare agents and the trans-fat and calorie-laden diets that are sold in impoverished communities.

When one considers morbidity and premature mortality, the source of the dangerous chemicals ingested matters little with respect to the final outcome. The only real difference is in the nature and mechanism of how they appear and the time involved before they manifest as pain, suffering, disease, and premature death. Clearly, trans-fats and high-calorie foods are ultimately as deadly as chemical warfare agents in their ultimate impact on society. This is especially true if poor communities are targeted for their distribution and sale.

Health care leaders must focus on the prevention of obesity rather than the treatment of the morbidities arising from it. Efforts at combating obesity that remain exclusively treatment focused will ultimately fail. This view applies to many of the issues encountered in the health care arena. Tobacco abuse, injury prevention, various infectious disease states, and many other health issues deserve this attention as well. However, I selected obesity to illustrate this point because of the tremendous implications for the future health and stability of this nation as a whole.

Addressing the obesity issue proactively is imperative; otherwise the impact of the medical, social, and financial costs will be difficult to withstand. In a population where over two-thirds of adults and one-third of children are overweight, there will not be enough health care workers or supportive service providers to care for an unhealthy and vastly obese population. The financial costs would be astronomical. In fact, to address this issue, the workforce itself would have to arise from within the population stricken with obesity.

Prevention must be the primary mechanism used to eliminate the potential for the development of morbidity and premature mortality related to obesity. A health and economic impact of such astounding proportions cannot be tolerated within our country or globally. Once again, a purely treatment-focused approach will ultimately fail.

In addition, the elimination of disparities must be combined with any attempts to increase community resilience against the aftermath of any man-made or natural occurrence or disaster. These occurrences are on the increase and are occurring against the backdrops of overpopulation, pollution, and poverty on a global scale.

On closer examination of this Theory of Social Disruption, it will become apparent that the existence of subpopulations of disparity weakens society as a whole. Their existence doesn't only weaken our social fabric locally but also threatens the general stability of society on a national and global scale. It is therefore imperative for this nation to provide the resources necessary to eliminate and rectify the root causes of disparities within all communities throughout the United States.

My hope is that this book, guided by my personal experiences as a physician, career military officer, and public official, will serve as an inspirational guide and catalyst for further insights and discoveries.

Above all, it should be used as an aid in the creation of actionable steps to protect and support the people of our great nation and the world. It is time for all of humanity to recognize that all humans are inextricably linked to a common future outcome within a global society.

PART 1

Theories About the Individual

Chapter 1

The Evolution of Human Adaptation, Perception, and Habituation

Surely, an understanding of human behavior and adaptation is central to understanding the human condition and its attendant needs. In this chapter, I will discuss three concepts I developed during my medical sciences training, while attending medical school. These concepts reflect my personal theoretical viewpoints. An understanding of the sequential development of human adaptation responses, sensory perceptions, and habitual behaviors are pivotal in creating public health programs that will succeed. These concepts merely represent potential ways of looking at how humans developed, individually and collectively, over the course of human evolution.

Always keep in mind that no model is capable of capturing this 'flame' called life or the essence of the human spirit. These conceptual models serve as a lens for looking at human adaptation, perception, and habituation over time and the implications for an individual as well as the collective community. Hopefully, they create a framework which aids the reader in the exploration of global human existence. I have provided some real-world experiences to illustrate how these concepts apply to everyday life.

I am not a mental health professional and defer to trained professionals the provision of accurate and complete information. My intent here is simply to provide a general framework I developed and find to be useful when approaching community-based intervention planning. It is not intended to diagnose or treat any behavioral or mental disorder. This then only serves as the launching point for self—and community-based exploration and discovery.

A Concept of Evolution and Adaptation

I once spoke to a coworker who was distraught over the death of her beloved parrot, which had died as a result of liver cancer. She felt guilty and responsible for the parrot's death, as she failed to detect the parrot's disease early enough to save its life. She lamented that if only she had been paying closer attention, her parrot would still be alive.

I explained that the parrot's death was not her fault. As a predator, the parrot tends to hide infirmities so as not to appear weakened. This instinct would protect it in the wild from becoming the next object of prey in the food chain. Her parrot's guise continued until it got to the proverbial 'end of its rope' and could no longer compensate for the presence of advanced disease—and the illness became apparent.

Human beings behave in a similar fashion, both consciously and subconsciously. The underlying, driving force is self-preservation. People may subconsciously ignore symptoms or consciously practice active denial. This is why preventing disease or detecting it and treating it early is so vitally important. These efforts help to move past potential shielding mechanisms before a person reaches and falls off the proverbial edge of a cliff. Nobody wants to end up like that parrot.

Prevention begins with the choices people continuously make throughout their lives. It is not just a matter of knowing the difference between *good* and *bad* choices; it is the actual choices consistently made. Clearly, a healthy diet forms the foundation of a healthy lifetime. Many people understand this and are able to provide healthy foods for their families. However, these choices are sometimes made for some communities without their active engagement in the process. This is typified by the creation and appearance of community-based 'food deserts.' These communities contain food sources of little or no nutritional value that may be directly harmful to humans.

When it is impossible to eat a healthy diet, people are forced into an unhealthy social paradigm that results in poor health. One must realize that this inequitable and unethical practice affects individuals, communities, and society as a whole. Food inequity leads to unnecessary and tragic health outcomes. To overcome this, those living in food deserts must participate in the food desert's eradication. Existing unhealthy food choices must be replaced by healthy food choices. These changes must affect every individual within the community.

People who live in food deserts develop coping mechanisms that can obscure the actual level of health-related damage within these communities. Much like the parrot that hid its infirmity, communities often appear healthier to the outsider than they truly are. The community members adapt to poor health outcomes that arise from poor diets and disrupted social circumstances. This occurs on the psychosocial level as well. The psychological defense mechanisms may cause a person to appear to be more resilient initially. However, when an individual decompensates beyond the breaking point, as noted with the parrot mentioned above, the results can be catastrophic.

These compensatory mechanisms give the false impression of individual and community stability. This can be reinforced by an overarching system external to the community that benefits from, and wishes to maintain, such a financially and politically expedient image. Some people profit from such relationships via the sale of their goods, even if they are innately unhealthy. Such a market system profits without accountability for the misfortunes in health outcomes encountered by the customers purchasing unhealthy products.

Community-based interventions must help people to recognize and remove these inadequate coping mechanisms. These coping mechanisms mask the true nature of the harmful situations within socially disrupted communities. When masks remain in place while health is compromised, this leads to social injustice, inequity, and disparate impacts. The underlying degrees of societal dysfunction and the inordinate occurrence of pain, suffering, and premature death are thus obscured. This creates dangerous spirals of masked morbidity and premature mortality that go unchecked—that is, until the measures that feign stability fail, and realities decompensate into readily apparent and disparate poor health outcomes.

Community-based interventions must recognize and carefully remove these masks. Confronting people with this removal of masks can be painful to them, so they must be approached with caution and care. These masks of adaptation may be regarded as conferring a degree of community member protection. Those who attempt to eliminate them may be perceived by community members as 'outsiders' attempting to overcome individual and community-based defense mechanisms.

On the other hand, these defenses prevent a true assessment of the injuries that have resulted from societal pressures that lead to social injustice, inequities, and the imposition of disparate impacts. In essence, these masks may offer some illusory degree of protection to the persons at risk. Yet their presence and persistence may block attempts to eradicate the social circumstances that give rise to the very need for these 'protective' masks within an unstable community environment.

Smoking is a good example of a protective mask a person might use to self-medicate. A smoker might think he or she looks 'cool' or believes smoking will 'settle the nerves' to deal with an underlying mental health issue, such as depression. Simply addressing smoking cessation may miss the mark because of the underlying link to depression, and the smoker's reliance upon the idea that smoking is beneficial at both social and personal levels.

Approaching smoking cessation as an isolated intervention step, without concern for these various social factors, might lead to a worsening of the underlying depression. It may also threaten to fragment the self-image of the individual involved. The removal of smoking as a coping mechanism might actually accelerate the behavior as well as miss the mark of its intended result: smoking cessation. A more prudent approach is to address smoking cessation with an appropriately staged and individualized intervention plan.

A New Concept Concerning Human Perception

Although many people ponder the potential existence of extrasensory perception (ESP), the senses one uses every day are truly remarkable. The following discussion represents a view I developed regarding the evolutionary trends guiding the progressive, sequential development of the senses. This conceptual framework offers a potential rationale for the sequential creation of the human senses over time. Although each of the senses is explained separately, they form part of a continuum with many overlapping periods.

It is important to note the co-evolutionary connections among the human senses, emotions, and cognitive abilities. These factors lead to a situation-based analysis, interpretation, and prediction regarding the natural and man-made phenomena that surround them. It also determines what an appropriate behavioral response should be. This process fundamentally determines individual and collective survival. My intent is to provide the reader with a view of how this process paves the way for the formulation and implementation of effective community interventions.

The Black Box

The human brain is encased within the bony box of the skull and has no direct contact with the outside world. Several sensory systems have been developed so the brain can gain information and conceptualize what the world outside this encasing black box is actually like. These sensory systems involve modalities such as touch, taste, smell, hearing, vision, and a sense of balance. Later, I will describe each of these in more detail within a conceptual framework I have developed.

This framework is an attempt to understand the purpose and need for the development of human sensory systems as they exist currently. It also sets the stage for a deeper understanding of what motivates humans at a very basic and profound level. As such, this discussion should be of some interest and assistance to community members and interventionists alike. One is less adept at addressing human issues when one does not comprehend the fundamental underpinnings of human existence and experience, and the related behavioral patterns that emerge.

The Sense of Touch

As organisms evolved through the millennia, the sense of touch developed as a response to threats or opportunities directly presented to an organism—that is, on an immediate and physical interaction level. For example, a one-celled organism responds to pH, temperature, and relative solvent gradients. It reacts to the immediate, tangible environment with attraction to or repulsion from an environmental agent, based upon the sensing of a potential benefit or harm, respectively.

Such a trend persisted as evolution proceeded to the appearance of multicellular organisms. The senses of balance and position also developed as we evolved to our current erect posture, guided by the effect of gravity and our relationship to the environment. Ultimately, the sensations of hot-cold, sharp-dull, wet-dry, and pressure on the skin gave rise to the experiential, emotion-based sensations of hunger, thirst, pleasure, pain, positioning, and balance. These sensations guided the development of human behaviors within the context of the natural environment. They offered a selective survival advantage for those who evolved to acquire these senses.

These sensations gave rise to the emotions, which control and guide physical responses to agents in the surrounding natural environment. Essentially, evolution moved from merely a physical level to a combined physical and emotional level. These emotions began to guide, through the establishment of behavioral patterns and responses, the physical outcomes within an environment.

Animals experienced the sensations of thirst and hunger, being guided by their emotions to seek water and food. The oral cavity became the portal for hydration, food energy acquisition, and breathing. These functions became essential to an organism's very survival.

The Sense of Taste

The sense of taste requires the proximate placement of a substance on the taste receptors. In humans, these taste receptors are located on the surface of the tongue. In order to taste something, it has to make direct contact with the receptors on the tongue. This is analogous to the direct contact required for touch, which necessitates the direct presentation of a physical stimulus, such as pressure, to perceive its presence.

Individuals have either a pleasurable or a negative reaction to the things they taste. A person will not eat what is repugnant in taste. This is part of the survival mechanism, which does not allow one to swallow things which are harmful, such as certain poisons and spoiled or contaminated food sources. Breathing and eating are essential for life. Taste is essential for obtaining a safe, reliable food source for energy.

The Sense of Smell

During this progressive evolution through physical and emotional levels of being, organisms developed the sense of smell. This was a tremendous leap forward. The sense of smell allowed for the first time the sensing of an environmental substance at a distance from the source of its production. Therefore, the environmental presence of a distant object could be detected without having to interact directly with it physically. Such interactions with distant objects could harbinger both benefits and risks of harm.

This new form of environmental perception also allowed for the emergence and development of what we experience as human consciousness. The aroma experienced had to be consciously tied to the object of the aroma's origin. This was then linked to the guiding forces of emotional states of being. The sense of smell requires the processing and interpretation of environmental agent stimulus inputs to arrive at correct behavioral response patterns. The sense of smell, by itself, is largely a two-dimensional, linear view of the world. The quality and relative intensity of the scent (concentration gradient) draws individuals toward or makes them move away from an external point source. This point source is the agent's point of origin, giving rise to the perceived smell.

The smell becomes more intense as one moves in the direction of the origin of the smell and less intense as one moves away. An individual may then have a tendency to move toward or away from a scent, such as that of a fruit orchard or smoke, respectively. The individual thereby secures a life-sustaining meal or avoids walking into a raging, life-threatening forest fire. This ability to selectively engage or avoid a distant object confers a selective survival advantage on those individuals able to interpret and use this stimulus to alter their behaviors appropriately.

The Sense of Hearing

The emergence of the sense of hearing provided environmental information from a more distant point than the sense of smell. The sense of hearing is based on the movement of energy waves through molecules and particles within the surrounding water or air. These energy waves form compression waves that give rise to perceived sounds. In addition, having two ears allows for the localization of the point of origin of a sound in three-dimensional space.

This is a selective survival advantage in that distant objects can be detected over a greater distance than with the sense of smell. Subsequently, the origin of a sound can be mapped out in three-dimensional space and either approached or avoided. It generally offers a greater degree of reaction time in response to a sound pattern. For instance, it could allow animals to hear a lion's roar in the distance. The emotion of fear would arise upon the perception of the sound of the roar. This would result in a classic 'fight or flight' response. This allows an animal to hold a defensive fighting stance, to freeze in place, 'playing dead,' or to flee to avoid an encounter that could result in injury or death. This also allowed for a sharper localization of the position of the roaring lion. Individuals began to map out their environments on a wider, three-dimensional level. The process was largely guided and aided by the emergence of higher consciousness. Conscious thought made possible the ability to conceptualize and attach significance to the origins of perceived sounds arising in a three-dimensional environment.

The sense of hearing is a tool for obtaining access to environmental resources that support the existence of life. For example, an individual could be drawn to the sound of a flowing river or waterfall when thirsty. This provides a selective survival advantage. The complex, intense, and often overpowering sounds encountered in modern times have dire consequences for those that dwell within noisy cities. Humans have not evolved to confront the sounds that have appeared over a relatively short evolutionary time span. These industrial-age sounds were not part of the natural evolutionary environment over multiple millennia.

The Sense of Vision

The development of sight dramatically enhanced the ability to interpret phenomena over a very long distance. Vision is an extraordinarily complex form of sensory perception. It relies on a series of complicated interactions with light energy-based stimuli. Like the sense of hearing, vision triggers both emotional responses as well as higher levels of conscious thought. Unscrupulous advertisers know this fact all too well.

Vision operates continuously during daylight and at night with the certain level of illumination necessary to support adapted night-time vision. Hearing operates intermittently in the natural environment, as its existence depends upon the physical production of sound waves. Sound wave production is generally not a continuous process in nature, unlike the urban environments we live in today. Light is also present in large amounts during the night in urban environments, unlike natural environments.

The development of vision allowed for the ability to conceptualize complex ideas and the creation of a drawing board of sorts to contemplate the world around us. I have often speculated whether the appearance of cave drawings was related to the realization of this newly acquired ability. The drawings themselves may have been an attempt to externalize and to explain to others the visions occurring within the mind of the drawer—that is, in the absence of a formalized language. It also engendered various aspects of the creative process, which mirrored human manipulations of the environments that surrounded them. Art in society today conveys cognitive ideas but also emotional content. Cave drawings were important in the development of communication skills, including languages as well as in the conveyance of ideas and emotional content.

The sense of vision has become a central component in most of our daily experiences in life. In modern society, the loss of vision has serious consequences for the affected person, despite the provision of disability support services and devices.

Vision and the Prediction of Future Events

Vision actually allows for a prolonged reaction time based upon the interpretation of visual information received from the environment. This often occurs over very long distances, almost instantaneously. Vision thereby permits one to make speculative, risk-based predictions of future incidents and events. This provides time to respond with corrective action prior to their predicted occurrences and anticipated consequences.

Vision allows for an increase in the amount of the allotted reaction time and a more calculated and strategic reaction to the anticipated occurrences. For instance, imagine that an individual is attempting to cross the street at a corner. This person then sees a speeding eighteen wheeler truck moving towards them down the road. Instinctively, the person jumps back from the truck's anticipated path in front of him—that is, prior to the truck even coming close to his body.

In effect, this person predicted that a dangerous and injurious situation would arise in the very near future were he not to alter and avoid his course of travel. He made a change in the course of travel based upon his prediction of the future.

This response to visual information regarding the anticipated outcome caused him to avoid possible injury or death. In effect, he used his cognitive ability to make a calculated prediction of future events and to make behavioral changes consistent with a better outcome. This individual consciously predicted, based on visual input, being struck by the truck if he were to proceed in the same manner. He then altered his behavior to avoid the previously predicted and negative potential outcome.

This takes a high level of contemplation and understanding of a risk-based and calculated prediction of future events on the part of the person involved. This leads to a heightened degree of survivability in an environmental setting. Survival is based on one's ability to analyze and make predictions of the future based upon an analysis of a current situation at a point in time. It also involves the ability to formulate and implement effective corrective action steps.

The Relationship Between Our Senses and the Cosmos

Combined with our cognitive abilities, our senses gave rise to an increasing ability on our part to predict the future. This also expanded the sphere of environmental space under human control. This is based upon an exploration and understanding of the natural and man-made components of the world and the surrounding universe.

Further, this understanding is the basis for a prediction of the consequences that would flow from an incident or event that is unfolding and being directly observed by an individual. Over time, these human observations have occurred from an increasingly distant vantage point. This has allowed an increased sphere of control and reaction time based upon a higher degree of cognitive functioning and the ability to predict potential outcomes. It has also resulted in a higher sense of physical and emotional security. That is, during this evolution through physical, emotional, and mental levels of being, humankind has sequentially developed the special human senses. The progressive addition of touch, taste, smell, hearing, and vision was associated with an ever-widening sense of our spatial environmental presence and our degree of control over our destiny.

There was a progression from direct physical contact to chemical gradient smell and taste recognition to mechanical particle-based sound wave recognition and finally to a visual, radiant-energy, light-based mode of perception. Therefore, there was a progressive movement from a solid, matter-based to a radiant energy-based form of perception for the recognition of external stimuli related to the surrounding natural environment over an ever-increasing distance. Humankind was able to touch rocks, yet also to perceive the moon, planets, and stars.

This may explain in part our historical need to explore planet Earth and our drive to explore the cosmos through space travel. Interestingly, during this evolutionary process, we also progressively moved from solid fuel sources, such as wood and coal, to the use of chemical petroleum-based fuels and then on to electrical and nuclear power sources. This represents a progressive move from matter-based to energy-based materials for use as fuel sources.

This has always been interesting to me in that humankind has progressed, as noted above, from physically-based to radiant energy-based modes of perception. Could this simply represent the extension of a human evolutionary drive to expand humankind's sphere of environmental presence and control? Are we attempting to satisfy our basic survival instincts and emotional needs for a sense of safety and control over our individual and collective destiny? Confronting the consequences of our collective and dire environmental impacts, we are now forced to pay closer attention, once again, to our immediate environments. The use of power sources based on photocells, solid hydrogen fuels, and wind power are now the focus of our attention.

There were many overlaps in the various stages of evolutionary development. They may represent a distinctive sequencing of environmental adaptations. There may be points where a collection of factors causes a developmental leap of the types noted by Eldredge and

Gould[1] in their theories of punctuated equilibrium, which were based on the earlier works of Mayr. Their works noted that there are periods in the paleontology-derived time records when, rather than having incremental changes, one encounters a marked shift in evolution. A particular characteristic changes rapidly over relatively few generations. This is followed by a period during which the characteristic is relatively stable and unchanged over vast amounts of time. This gives rise to the term 'punctuated equilibrium,' as one views this repetitive pattern upon examination of paleontological records over an expansive period.

I speculate that the appearance of certain environmental factors and developmental features in specific combinations may have been synergistic or inhibitory in their ability to foster the occurrence of further physical evolutionary changes. This would potentially result in the occurrence of more rapidly realized evolutionary changes with respect to their appearance or disappearance within the environment. However, if one were to apply this concept to emotional, mental, and spiritual evolutionary development, would each of these have their own innate periodicity with respect to a punctuated equilibrium viewpoint?

Additionally, are there periods during which these physical, emotional, mental, and spiritual states of being are more or less aligned or even asynchronous? Are they supportive or in conflict with our individual and collective survival? For instance, one may possess the mental ability to work with atomic energy and yet have the spiritual and emotional adeptness of a cave person when constructing and using an atomic weapon. If collective survival is the stated goal of a society, why do we pollute the environment and have wars? If individual and collective survival are so important to us, why do we participate in self-destructive behaviors?

Nonetheless, despite the preceding questions, these adaptations progressively gave us greater control over our interactions with the environment. In part this was an attempt to

---

[1]   Stephen Jay Gould and Niles Eldredge, "Punctuated Equilibria: The tempo and mode of evolution reconsidered," *Paleobiology* 3, (1972): 115-151.

create a higher sense of individual and collective stability and security. With more control over the environment, we could then feel more secure on both a personal and a collective level. However, what should come with this is a sense of interpersonal and environmental responsibility. Accordingly, this must be based upon the correct ethical and moral principles aimed at individual health, environmental sustainability, and global peace.

It is also important to note that the world is moving at an ever-increasing pace. This pace has demanded humans to react with ever-increasing speed and accuracy with respect to information inputs and outputs. This is sometimes associated with the cost of a resulting poor health outcome. Such a vantage point would appear to be in contradistinction to the concept of survival I have noted concerning human evolution.

The theory I have posed stresses that the evolutionary drive tends to increase both the time available to react to a situation and the feelings of control over a situation over greater distances. I have concerns over whether information technology trends attempting to 'bring people closer together' are actually moving against the evolutionary trend of establishing a sense of individual security and safety. Are we creating problems for human existence through the imposition of such a social policy? From this standpoint, is this policy of media globalization fundamentally flawed, leaving little time for human adaptation responses to its potential impacts? Is society creating social policies guided by the viewpoint that 'faster, more, and bigger is better while neglecting to recognize the fundamental human need for survival, security, self-control, and self-determination?

The Schism Between the Emotions and the Mind

In my view, at some point there was a movement, in part, away from an emotionally directed behavioral pattern to one that relies on higher cognitive control. I also conjecture that this resulted in a schism that arose between the emotional and the mental states of being. In essence, the potential sources of control—the emotional and the mental—vied for control of behavioral patterns. The mind and the emotions battle continuously for the ultimate control over an individual's physically based destiny.

There has been an ever-present and continuous battle between our earlier developed emotional mechanisms and our more recently emergent higher consciousness. As they vie for the control of our physical self, it must be appreciated that neither the emotional nor the mental state should be allowed to be preeminent, as both are required for a healthy life. The existing balance between these for resolving any given issue is all too important.

I propose that the discrepancies arising from this battle between our emotional and cognitive selves, when vying for control over our physical self, gives rise to the origins of anxiety and stress. They also tend to exacerbate any underlying, extrinsically imposed, or innate degree of mental disorder. Since these are cognitively based perceptions of reality, rather than those originating in physically based experiences, such as sharp and dull sensations, they are experienced in a different way. That is, they may result in feelings such as discomfort, depression, emotional pain, rage, or anger.

Our emotional self was directly tied to earlier, physical modes of sensory perception. It now has to deal with thoughts, interpretations, and ideas arising from our cognitive self. The emotional self may as a result have great difficulties in interpreting and dealing with these thoughts. These socially contrived thoughts do not arise from the physical platform the nervous system initially evolved to deal with, which was largely guided by emotional engagement.

Note that students may stay up all night to finish a term paper, neglecting eating, sleeping, and even going to the bathroom. The student's mental state suppresses her emotional responses, which are a reaction to what her physical state is experiencing as discomfort or even pain. In this case, the mind rules over the emotions and subjects her body to a high degree of physical discomfort in order to complete what her mind has set out to do—finish the term paper. Of course, this is at the expense of meeting her physical as well as emotional needs. This can result in physical discomfort, anxiety, stress, and even depression as a consequence of the application of an overriding degree of mental control. The result is a direct physical impact under the guidance of an overriding mental control mechanism.

As noted, psychological consequences also occur and can deliver a psychosomatic and emotional payload as well. A response to this physical and emotional burden may be the development of harmful compensatory mechanisms. For example, compensatory coping behaviors such as excessive caffeine or alcohol consumption, overeating, and smoking may arise in the lives of these students. This may represent an emotional regression to the oral stage of development, when the taste sensation needed to be satisfied. The more proximate application of agents that give rise to sensory stimuli at the level of the tongue may be providing comfort to the emotional state at a very basic proximate level. This is then interpreted as security, comfort, satisfaction, and self-control by the individual at an emotional level. In essence it is a retreat from the more expansive and unpredictable environment.

I will describe this in greater detail throughout the book with respect to the mouth being the 'gateway' for the vast majority of chronic diseases. Note that addictions have a focal point in the mouth, which can lead to food, alcohol, tobacco, illicit drug, and legal medication abuse. The mouth may also serve as the portal of entry for sexually transmitted infections and poisons such as lead. The introduction of these substances into one's body is largely guided by how and if one uses their hands to bring them to the mouth. Of course the hand is only responding to signals from both the mental and emotional states of being, which struggle over the control of the physical self.

On the other hand, if there is a positive relationship between our emotions and our conscious experiences, one will have the positive experience of joy or heightened self-esteem. In fact, I speculate that the sense of spirituality and that of compassion are exact expressions of a very high level of integration and cohesion between emotional and mental states of being. We may find this being physically expressed through creative acts such as meditation, singing, dancing, painting, or playing a musical instrument. This is also why there may be a tendency to turn to these activities for relief from the stresses caused by persistent and unresolved mental and emotional control schisms and imbalances.

People intellectually understand why it is necessary to avoid the catastrophic consequences stemming from standing in front of a speeding eighteen-wheeler. Then why do they ignore what their hand has brought to their mouth when it results in disease or a poor health outcome?

The Silent Gray Serpent

The vast majority of people in America routinely ignore the consequences of their health-related behaviors. This may have to do both with the relative immediacy as well as the lack of a full comprehension of the expected negative health effects. In the *Black Swan*, which I recommend you read, Nassim Taleb does an excellent job of noting the impact of the occurrence of low-probability, high-impact events.[2]

In considering the concept I am speaking of here, I would like to call this phenomenon the Silent Gray Serpent. This is the concept of a high probability and delayed high-impact event. For example, if a person were living in a food desert, it might be difficult, if not impossible, for him to get a healthy selection of foods. Therefore, there is a very high probability that he will ingest unhealthy products, as they are the only ones available to satisfy his hunger. If there is a delay in the onset of morbidity and premature mortality expected or envisioned by participating in this self-destructive behavior, there may be little incentive for him to change his behavior.

As time progresses, however, there is also a high impact price to pay as ill health associated with pain, suffering, and the chances for a premature mortality begin to take the stage. This is the appearance of the Silent Gray Serpent in his life. Silently and progressively, the

---

2   Nassim Nicholas Taleb, *The Black Swan* (New York: Random House, 2007).

effects of his underlying, unhealthy behaviors destroy his chances for a healthy, happy, and long life.

As I note in later chapters, the ripple effects of the silent gray serpent extend outward to affect one's family, workplace, and community. As individuals succumb to the consequences of poor health and the side effects of social and fiscal instability, the persons they are associated with will be impacted as well. However, I do not wish to imply that one has to 'turn gray' to suffer the consequences of poor health. Poor health outcomes certainly can occur very early in life, as with childhood type 2 diabetes. The gray only implies the need for a passage of a requisite period of time (latency period) over which one participates in the unhealthy behavior before it manifests itself as injury, illness, or disease. Once again, it does not imply that one's hair must turn gray before the consequences materialize.

This phenomenon also occurs at a population-based level. Essentially all the individuals in a disparately impacted community are exposed to the poor sources of nutrition within a food desert environment. This portends the development of an entire community stricken with the effects of poor health and a shortened life span.

The Drive to Self-Medicate and the Process of Adaptation

With respect to unhealthy behaviors, an individual may also be driven by attempts at self-medication. This tendency to self-medicate is an attempt to satisfy emotionally, an underlying source of internal conflict. The source of the conflict may be of internal or external origin and causes distress and pain. This is recognized at physical, emotional, mental, and even spiritual levels. The unhealthy behavior occurring without an immediate impact seems to offer a viable solution for this need to be met at the time. However, one ultimately pays the Silent Gray Serpent price for this behavior.

There is also the prospect that a natural tendency toward adaptation may make it more difficult to discern a progressive decline in one's health status. This is especially true should this process occur over a prolonged period. The individual then slowly adapts to a progressively worsening health status. This slow decline in health may not be recognized by that person. Even if her health is grossly abnormal, it may not be apparent, or even a concern, to her. Additionally, a family or group may support her self-destructive behavior. This can actually hasten the person's health status decline. This is why it is critical to have appropriately trained mental health professionals intimately involved in community health intervention planning and operations. Mental health and social work professionals are worth their weight in gold, and they should be supported and utilized.

The Denial of Recognition for Intellectual Worth

The rates of physical, emotional, mental, and spiritual development vary. This is true regardless of whether one looks at an individual person or a community as a whole. Many times, individuals are denied access to the resources required to bring into fruition their hopes, dreams, and creativity.

If a person is denied his right to express his skills, talents, and abilities through the recognition of his worth as a cognitively based and intellectually functional human being, he is deeply harmed. He will react from an emotional level, having been denied the requisite recognition of his worth as a mentally competent and fully functional participant in society.

This has tremendous implications for those who are disparately impacted by social messaging and a lack of resources for both cognitive development and achievement. Societal and institutional practices that strip them of this recognition constantly further compound this impact.

This fosters the creation of pockets of individuals that are socially disruptive. Those having been socially disenfranchised from their innate talents, abilities, skills, inner dreams, hopes, and aspirations for the future by society at large will react from an emotional vantage point. This is a result of the stripping away of their ability to provide cognitive input and control that is recognized to be plausible and valid. This is a tragic injustice to any human being and to society as a whole. Frankly, it is tantamount to physical, emotional, intellectual, and spiritual murder.

The longer we deny the existence of such social influences and injustices, the worse this source of social disruption will become. Attempts to fix this through social planning schemes that exclude community participation and fail to address this most basic view of the origin of the problem will ultimately fail. Indeed, such attempts will provide more destructive input than constructive assistance in attempting to resolve the problem. This is especially true if there is a conscious and explicit lack of recognition of the true underlying causes of the problems. Such a denial of the existence and root causes for poor social conditions further exacerbates the problem. Failure to recognize community involvement and input from the viewpoint of those in need is a tragic mistake. Such an approach can lead to more harm than good.

The Concept of Habituation

There is also the effect of habituation, in which one develops repetitive behavioral patterns that give rise to both positive and negative consequences. For example, envision a caveman holding a large club and standing just inside the opening of a dimly lit cave. An angry bear then enters the cave, and the caveman immediately strikes it with the club, knocking it unconscious. This is a good thing for the caveman.

Next a tiger enters the cave, and he repeats his actions, knocking it unconscious. This action is also good for the caveman. After multiple repetitions, this becomes a basically good and automatically occurring action on the caveman's part; he is protecting himself. Subsequently, however, another animal enters the cave, and he instinctively and automatically repeats his action with skill and speed, knocking it unconscious. But then he looks down and discovers that he has knocked out his pet dog. Thus, the process of responding to things in a repetitive, habitual way can also result in negative consequences.

In the modern world, habitual behavioral patterns can have good results. Habits such as brushing one's teeth in the morning or putting on a seat belt in a car have very positive benefits. These habitual acts can result in the creation of subconscious behaviors as well. For example, a person can drive to work and not remember exactly how she got there. She cannot recall all the steps taken to arrive there when consciously reflecting upon the course of the trip to work. She does not remember stopping and obeying the traffic signals or observing safe-distance rules while driving. Despite this, her mind and body was coordinated enough to get her safely to work without the need for conscious recognition of the details on how this was accomplished.

Consider trying this exercise: spell out loud the following series of words as they are presented below, in order. Then turn the page. As quickly as possible, answer the question that appears at the top of the page.

The first word is CROP.

The next word is DROP.

The next word is MOP.

The next word is COP.

The next word is DROP.

The next word is CROP.

The next word is TOP.

The next word is CROP.

Now turn the page.

COL. *Damon T. Arnold, M.D., M.P.H.*

When you get to a green light, what do you do?

Try this with friends too.

Here is what happens: the readers are participating in a conditioning exercise in which they parallel process thoughts in their brain. Human beings are hard-wired to conserve energy both on a physical as well as mental level. Therefore, they seek answers that seem familiar after being conditioned, which tend to conserve mental energy. Chances are if they performed the task correctly, they said and may have spelled the word *stop*. Of course, the correct answer is to *go*. On the physical level, this is why people have to change their exercise routine on a regular basis to get the same benefit. Humans are very adaptable, and this is just one facet of adaptability.

As people participate in routine behaviors throughout the day, they use relatively little conscious recognition of the steps involved in the completion of routine tasks. In fact, on the subconscious level, they habitually stop at all the traffic signals and stop signs while driving to work without conscious recognition of their presence. However, habituation can also result in harmful consequences, such as occurs with smoking, drug addiction, and overeating. Eating one potato chip may be fine, but eating a whole bag often can be disastrous for one's health. Once again, behavioral patterns are shaped by and arise from adaptations to outside influences, whether on an emotional or cognitive level. This depends upon how one mentally and emotionally deals with his or her perceptions of and reactions to the environment he or she lives in.

Human beings become more energy efficient when presented with repetitive tasks to complete. The exercise becomes easier over time. The conditioned person then has to change her routine to get the same effects as earlier. Note that this form of conditioning, as in the above example, can occur in seconds. Further, contemplate what can happen to a person after years of exposure to negative thoughts about herself, encountered in society over a lifetime. Societal statements indicating that she is not smart enough, fast enough, or of the right gender, age, or racial background can have devastating consequences for an individual. This can be a very destructive process for the person, who begins to believe the information presented about herself, even if it is not at all true. It can be internalized and happen on a subconscious as well as conscious level.

Dogmatic thinking occurs in a similar fashion. This is where an individual believes that what he thinks to be true is indeed true—even if it is not a valid viewpoint. The fear of being found to be wrong outweighs the possible delight of finding the valid answer. This can block further progress as one blindly and erroneously stakes out the claim of knowing 'the correct answer.' Such a dogmatic thinker is essentially unwilling to change his viewpoint due to the fear engendered by the underlying insecurities of a potential loss of self-worth.

A person who constantly participates in destructive behaviors raises the risk of developing physical pain, suffering, and a premature death. However, he or she must also live with the consequences as well. The repercussions also extend to his or her family members, friends, coworkers, and society as a whole. The ripple effects can have staggering consequences throughout his or her social network. The key here is to recognize, defuse, and deal with the elimination of these destructive patterns that all community members live with to one degree or another. Cycles of societal disruptions leading to unhealthy outcomes must be broken and replaced with behavioral patterns leading to healthy outcomes at all levels of society.

Your Relationship to the Community

Carl Jung, a protégé of Sigmund Freud, spoke of a collective consciousness within society. The ability to think and the attempt to construct a framework of reality for defining human existence has created the need for interpersonal communication. In response to this need, humankind developed the capacity for creating symbolisms and languages. Various ideas and concepts were thrown about and resulted in the collective way humans think within a society and its various, distinctive subcultures.

There are many languages and subcultures globally. A high degree of diversity can also occur on the same city block with current levels of globalization and travel. From just such a community crucible arise the collective cultural practices and ideologies of a society's members. With the exchange of information comes a risk of miscommunication leading to false impressions, the creation of myths, and the formation of invalid opinions of others. This can go further to result in the creation of dogma and destructive ideologies—regardless of their invalidity and any potential harm they may impose upon the members of a community. Despite this, they nevertheless are incorporated into a culture's belief system and practices over time.

Conversely, positive and appropriate communication can result in constructive ideologies directed at supporting the health and well-being of community members. Such ideologies have significance and meaning for the members of the culture or subculture they arise within and are a part of. Eventually, they can become entrenched within the community, forming the basis for ritualistic, habitual behaviors that lead to healthy outcomes and are reinforced over time.

This process shapes the way one thinks about life and the views that he or she forms in reaction to existing community factors or outside interventions within his or her life space. For example, a person may sit down to eat a high-calorie, fat-laden meal, followed by several alcoholic drinks and a cigarette. Obviously none of these activities are healthy. However, these acts may be done in the context of a traditional Thanksgiving meal, where overeating, drinking alcohol, and smoking by family members are condoned as acceptable behaviors during the holidays.

For any intervention to work there must first be an understanding of the culture it is to be inserted in. The behaviors that already exist there—from the community member's viewpoint, not from the interventionist's—must be clearly and fully understood.

The interpretation of whether it makes 'good and logical' sense for community members to participate in an identified 'negative' behavior must take into account the views of the community members themselves.

Cultural anthropologists have recognized this for decades and offer keen insights on this point of view with respect to community-based interactions.

In addition, note the term 'good and logical.' Despite our attempt to remain objective, our subjective views and values will always be a part of the objective, logic-driven analysis process—on both the conscious and the subconscious levels. Overzealous attachment to one's unwavering viewpoints without a degree of flexibility will result in a failed intervention strategy and can possibly result in harm to those one seeks to assist.

Leave the Stereotypes Behind

On many of my military missions, both within the continental United States and abroad to Africa, Central and South America, and the Middle East, I learned the following lessons. One cannot simply assume that his or her understanding or assigned value placed upon specific issues are the same as those held by the community members themselves. The collection of data is an attempt to characterize community-based dynamics and offers only a snapshot of the reality. However, the underlying beliefs and experiences of community members carry much greater weight than pure data when attempting to create a valid, accurate, and comprehensive understanding of the needs of the community being served.

The viewpoints of community members have many implications for how they chose to structure their environments and protect what they have come to treasure in life. If an interventionist's first principle is to do no harm, then he or she must not impose judgments, which are often based on erroneous, stereotypical viewpoints.

If one attempts to insert an intervention with an incorrect form of delivery, due to a lack of truly understanding the community, it can have disastrous results. It may also alienate the community members from those attempting to provide service to them.

Cultural and linguistic sensitivities must be kept in mind within the context of any proposed or existing intervention strategy. Once again, both cultural and linguistic competency must be kept in mind when intervening. Further, one must decipher his or her own beliefs and intentions in attempting to implement the intervention in the first place. What is your motive? What are you getting out of it? What are you really giving the community members? Have you attempted to assist or to control community members? Get to know who they truly are and what they truly want and need.

Engaging Community Members as True Partners

There needs to be a concerted effort to train and educate the community members themselves for participation in the intervention process. Always remember, that there is an implied sense of helplessness imparted to community members who eventually perceive their selves to be the recipients of outside help.

This is particularly true when they are not included in planning, decision making, and actual implementation of the specific services being offered and put into operation. For these community members, this sense of helplessness can reside at the emotional level and arise from a reaction to an external, institutionally imposed sense of inadequacy and demoralization. They essentially feel helpless and unable to provide the solutions to their own problems themselves. To overcome this externally imposed negativity, they must feel and truly be empowered to be full participants in any community healing process.

It is also true that one cannot form a true connection with community members if they are viewed as outsiders. To influence the behaviors and actions of others to any significant degree, one must forge an emotional and mental alignment with them. The interventionist cannot supplant the essence and the right to self-determination of an individual with a construct he or she feels the person should emulate. Community members must feel respected and accepted for who they are. One has to persuade them that better options exist for them to have a healthier and happier lifetime.

All communications, whether written or spoken, should be viewed through the community's eyes before distribution and implementation. Community members must also have the final word on the acceptance of an intervention strategy. Cultural and linguistic sensitivity are essential for effective communication and messaging to occur.

Interventionists bring multiple images of themselves with them into any space they choose to enter. There are personal identifiers such as race, ethnicity, age, gender, clothing, personal habits, language, and even the music listened to. These attributes give rise to the impressions that others will form of who the interventionist is as an individual. However, this may be distinctly different from the impression an interventionist may have of himself or herself. Needless to say, every person has several valid and invalid, negative or positive views of his or her 'authentic self.'

In addition, one's degree of self-discipline, drive, and capacity to form meaningful and satisfying relationships are crucial to the intervention process. This also aids an interventionist's efforts in crossing the usual divides and boundaries of organizational, professional, and community-based cultural associations. Awareness and connectivity within the community is essential for one to accomplish the bridging of these entities. In forming these relationships, one's first allies are the people one is helping. This is true even if this is the very culture one has always been a part of. It is important to realize that relationships and trust are developed and modified over time.

The perceptions various community members have of themselves as well as of the interventionist will change. The direction and form these relationships will take depends upon the relative successes or failures of these social interactions. It is important to realize that one's personal integrity, a sense of compassion, and attitude are extremely important in the establishment of trusting relationships. An interventionist must frequently reflect upon these in his or her 'personal mirror' and develop them in a positive direction.

COL. *Damon T. Arnold, M.D., M.P.H.*

Lead by Example with Competence, Passion, and Compassion

The foregoing challenges require curiosity, courage, motivation, and the development of social skills. The authority one carries with a title allows a certain degree of process control. This includes the leveraging of resources. This must be accompanied by the ability to influence the creation of, and to be in compliance with, effective and best practices-based intervention strategies.

Both the intervention team members and those who are to be the recipients of these efforts must understand the relevance and importance of demonstrating the effectiveness of an intervention strategy. One must combine passion with compassion every step along the way. Interventionists must also recognize that they do not have all the answers and will gain much more than they are able to give. Let metrics, competencies, and compassion for community members gauge the degree to which one is affecting a positive change in the lives of those served. The final verdict of success, however, is to be determined by the community members themselves.

It is important to understand human behavior, to develop relationship networks with people, and to recognize the networks already in existence within the community. Essentially, one must become the type of person people want to listen to and place within their circle of trust.

In the next chapter, I will discuss how one's personal actions determine his or her health care destiny as well as the concept of a societal health gradient. These form the underlying framework in which behavioral choices are made on a daily basis and set the stage for the theory of social disruption.

Chapter 2

Your Hand Determines Your Health Care Destiny

One must recognize the actual origins of poor health outcomes. The leading causes of pain, suffering, and premature death are diseases and injuries, which are almost always preventable. People often equate the occurrences of disease and illness with natural phenomena, such as bad weather or earthquakes. That is, it is assumed that they are completely out of our control and due to externally imposed misfortunes. However, the truth is that diseases are most often inflicted by a single instrument: *one's own hand*. Hold your hand up before your face and look at it closely. Behold the 'instrument' of your health outcome 'destiny.' Unhealthy practices are the cause for the vast majority of health care outcomes that end in chronic disease.

I will now intentionally focus on you, the interventionist, in a more personal way. I hope to challenge you to confront your own health practices and to walk the walk of what you preach.

Your Hand Determines Your Future

Perhaps the term *destiny* mistakenly implies the advent of an unforeseeable, uncontrollable outcome. Destiny flows not as a matter of chance but as a matter of the choices a person makes. This touches exactly upon the point I wish to make. The 'outcome' lies in your ability to correctly respond to environmental cues that are directed toward a healthy outcome rather than an unhealthy one. In many ways, your hand determines your destiny through your behavior. For example, your hand can be used to increase personal and societal stability or to impose a greater degree of personal and societal disruption. In fact, with respect to the development of the vast majority of the societal chronic disease burdens and premature deaths, your own hand plays the major role.

There are several self-destructive and socially destructive acts you can participate in with your hands. I have told patients for over three decades now that the mouth is the gateway for the cause of over 90 percent of chronic illnesses and diseases. What you put into your mouth largely determines what your self-inflicted disease burden will become. This includes the use of food (harmful types or amounts), chewing or smoking tobacco, illegal drugs, inappropriate legal medication usage, or excessive amounts of drinking alcohol. The old saying 'pick your poison' is a literal statement of fact when it comes to choices that lead to a poor health outcome.

This is the basis for the Silent Gray Serpent phenomenon I alluded to in the first chapter. The ingestion of these substances is followed by the delayed onset of a poor health outcome, with pain, suffering, and a premature death as its calling cards.

The hand can also be used to inflict violence in the form of a fist or to pull the trigger of a weapon. However, the negative outcomes stemming from acts of commission, what you do with your hand, can also arise from acts of omission, what you neglect to do with your hand. For instance, you can correctly avoid using your hand to over eat bad things yet fail to use your hand to eat healthy foods. Not using your hand to do things that have a stabilizing, positive outcome can, therefore, have devastating consequences for your future health and well-being. This includes avoiding things such as wearing a seat belt while driving. It also includes not opening a workout facility door for exercise or a clinic door for preventive health evaluations and appropriate early medical intervention. Also, not putting on a condom before sexual intercourse is extremely dangerous in the current social climate.

If you do not wash your hands before preparing food or improperly store prepared foods, you can experience an episode of food poisoning.

The bacteria you introduce due to improper food handling can produce toxins and or multiply in food. You can also shake hands or sneeze into your hand and spread bacterial and viral infections.

Your hand can also be used to cover your eyes from the sight of social injustices and violent behaviors that inflict harm upon other people. It can also cover your mouth, keeping you from speaking up against and reporting injustice and violence. This is a responsibility of everyone, including you.

Your Hand Is Under the Control of Your Personal Behavior

Of course, your personal behavior controls your hand. As discussed earlier, this is based on conscious and subconscious thoughts and emotions that lead to the actions you take. Be careful not to participate in self-destructive acts or destructive acts directed against others. The consequences of these decisions flow from your behaviors, based upon the personal choices you make.

Many times the schism between the mind and the emotions results in such states as depression and self-destructive acts. This can serve as the point of origin for behaviors such as self-medication and suicide. Depression can result in overeating that leads to obesity and physical disease. In essence, food serves to satiate emotional pain, stress, and anxiety to some degree.

It is important to seek help in these situations and to take steps to change your behaviors. This can literally make the difference not only between your happiness and sadness but between life and death. There are many ways to get help in this regard.

Depression is probably the most common disorder in society and can be effectively treated in the vast majority of cases. If you need help, get it. It is very often due to, or worsened by, social situations that you are immersed in. The important thing is that you can and must overcome bad outcomes by taking appropriate actions. This includes eliminating those things that inflict harm upon you.

Remember, whatever your circumstances, you are a miraculous human being and deserve a physically, emotionally, mentally, and spiritually healthy, and pain-free, happy life. Only you ultimately have the power and the ability to determine this good outcome for yourself. If you are attempting to help others with this, you need to do this for yourself first. Not only is it important for you to lead by example, but you must also recognize the potential for carrying your own unresolved issues into the community you wish to support with services.

The hand can also be extended to create friendships and acts of peace. It can console those who are distraught, wipe away tears, repair broken hearts, and be used for meditation and prayer. Every human being has the power and the ability to determine that the best possible outcome will occur for them.

Once you understand the relationship between your behavior and your personal health outcome, you can take affirmative steps to ensure a better and healthy future—that is, by choosing to use your hand to participate in healthy behaviors.

The Social Determinants of Health and the Societal Health Gradient

The social determinants of health are based upon genetic factors, social nurturing, and the geopolitical situation an individual finds himself or herself in. The conditions under which one is born, works, lives, and ages have direct impacts on how one's health outcome will unfold.

The distribution of money, social power, resources, environmental conditions, and social policies and circumstances largely determines where one is found along the scale of what I have termed the societal health gradient. This societal health gradient must be viewed as a continuous spectrum that extends from the extremes of good health to poor health, as they are distributed within a population in a designated geographic location. It also yields a comprehensive snapshot of the situation one finds oneself in at any point in time. It is fluid and dynamic.

There are many factors that impact each of us on a daily basis and in a multitude of ways. To a large extent, these factors determine what our short-term and long-term health outcomes will be. I will explain the importance of this health gradient in greater detail in subsequent chapters.

Chapter 3
The Relationship That Dwells Within

Constantly, we, as humans, are on a search for greater meaning in life. During times of upheaval and change, there is always a period of fear and discomfort when people face the unknown. This is directly related to our relationship with the universe that surrounds us. The prospect of change or of approaching a new horizon for the development of a new vision of what it means to be human is exciting, but it's unsettling at the same time. When we live during times of change, there is always a period of fear and discomfort as we face the unknown. We experience a sense of loss of control over our direction and destination.

There are several coexistent dimensions with respect to the human experience within our community settings. Some of these are based upon our sense of purpose and orientation toward the community's social environment. Other societal issues may be more complex and difficult to fathom. Despite this, humans attempt to adjust to societal pressures. In fact, our very survival continuously depends on our ability to order and maneuver the environment that surrounds us. This occurs on the physical, emotional, mental, and spiritual levels simultaneously.

Most systems tend to be supportive and beneficial. However, like cancer in a body, some dysfunctional, pervasive, persistent, and self-destructive social ideologies and systems result in a tendency toward social disruption. The hallmarks of their existence are in the forms of observable pain, suffering, and premature death among community members afflicted by their impacts. The goal is to eliminate what causes these circumstances to occur. However, the approach to these external issues begins with what dwells within us. To that end, this section opens an inwardly directed door.

The Focus Within

I have been practicing martial arts for many years. This chapter contains several stories that will shed some light on the dynamic process of self-realization. I present them for you to read. One story is of ancient origin, and I modified it. The other is of my own creation. You should reflect upon how they are present within your own life and hopefully apply them when needed.

The Goal and the Ego

I created the following story some years ago. It is about one of my experiences in the martial arts.

> A prospective student walked in front of a martial arts master. The master asked what the visit concerned. The student explained that his goal was to be a master martial artist as well. The would-be student then picked up a long staff used for armed combat. The master immediately produced a like staff, which materialized instantly, startling the prospective student. The master used it to knock the staff from the prospective student's hand with a single, swift blow.
>
> The student was amazed but perplexed at the same time and asked, *"Why master did you strike the staff from my hand?"*
>
> The master gazed deeply into the student's eyes and replied, *"By picking up the staff and confronting me, you signified that you have already attained the goal of mastering the staff as a weapon."* The master then went on to explain that the first thing for the student to realize is that the staff is merely an inanimate extension of his 'self.' The master noted that the staff could be only as strong as what he has mastered within his 'self.' *"You cannot walk in the light of the goal of self-mastery if you have not yet achieved it, or the realities of adversity will teach you the lessons of a lack of preparation."*

The student then asked if he was accepted as a student by the master martial artist. The master smiled and said, *"I have already given you the most important lesson there is to learn."* The master then posed this question to the student, *"You have much to teach yourself. Do you accept yourself as a student?"*

The first step in making any change is to recognize the need for acquiring the skills required to get to your goal. This may involve overcoming a denial of the need to acquire them and the recognition that their acquisition is essential for a positive, healthy, and fulfilling life as you envision it. The first instructor of any art lies completely within you. You must take the first step by committing to action upon the path of self-discovery.

The Martial Arts Zen Masters

The next story is ancient and was conveyed to me by word of mouth during my childhood. I have not been able to find the original text or author and only paraphrase what I heard orally decades ago. I have added a bit to the story as I think it applies to the situation facing people who are considering changing their behaviors. Hopefully, this will help you as you change your habits to attain a healthier life.

There once were two martial arts Zen masters who were walking upon a dirt road. They both were dressed in full martial arts regalia, with swords within their respective sheaths. There was a full moon at the end of the path that night. Pine trees lined both sides of the road. Lightning bugs blinked throughout the trees and blended with the twinkling stars above to form an arc of light that surrounded the pathway.

As they walked down the road together, one martial arts master turned his head to ask the other a question. *"Master, tell me, when two ferocious tigers face each other in heated battle and conflict, what is the result?"* The other master did not even utter a sound, and they continued to walk down the road together.

39

> After the two masters had walked another two miles, the master turned his head and said, "Master, when two ferocious tigers face each other in heated battle and conflict, one of the tigers will be irreparably harmed. It will be maimed and live out the rest of its days in utter misery and pain." The master took another two steps, turned his head again, and said, "And the other one will die!"

This is a very powerful story. At first glance it may seem to be a simple story about two tigers fighting. Over time, I have given this story several interpretations. The one that I feel is appropriate here is that the two masters represent a balanced harmony between two opposing but complementary forces that have learned to live in harmony.

You see, you have forces within yourself that sometimes work together and sometimes against each other. One force says you are gifted, and the other says you are worthless. We all have a tendency to fight within and against ourselves in so many ways. We have to learn to accept our weaknesses and occasional lapses in judgment as we learn to be better without beating ourselves up too badly. The reality is that you possess many talents, abilities, skills, and positive attributes that are within a framework that is ultimately human. As these qualities develop within your being, be persistent yet patient and compassionate with yourself.

It is not that either force is necessarily good or bad. Rather, they both are absolutely required and essential for you to be a whole individual. But the balancing of them should be in an ever-increasing positive direction with respect to your health and state of being. This must be accomplished while still being compassionate and supportive of your efforts and yourself as you seek to change. This approach should ultimately increase your compassion for others as well, as they develop and meet their challenges, defeats, and successes.

Unlike the tigers fighting, we must learn not to stick the claws that maim or kill into ourselves or into others. To participate in such negative activities is very *self*-destructive and can result in us not accomplishing our goals. It also supports the existence of social disruption, which directly impacts each of us as individuals and extends into the lives of those surrounding us. We must move toward perfecting what it means to be human.

Make sure to get the exercise you need, as this can help to reduce stress and improve your mood. You may engage in several activities that help to reduce your stress levels and put you in a proper frame of mind to address your personal and social circumstance. There are classes offered with respect to meditation, yoga, and the martial arts, including Tai Chi, which can be of great assistance in this process. I coined the word *medipraytion* many years ago as a focal point for the combination of a deeply meditative state combined with a prayerful state of being.

You must devise your own routine for reducing stress and combatting the negative emotions and physical consequences that arise within the context of our current societal structures. I have listed several resources to assist you in this process in the resources sections of this book.

It continues to astound me that the educational system does not provide instruction, to my knowledge, at any level of education on how to live, to be healthy, and to seek a happy, stress-free existence. This seems to me to be a fundamental lesson to teach students as they progress through the educational system. It also represents a fundamental flaw in Western thought on how one should develop a society directed to benefitting the health and well-being of its members.

A Perspective on Aging

When I was in high school, college, and medical school, I wrote many poems. I would like to share two of them with you. The first has to do with the impressions I had after seeing the care provided to senior citizens in austere health care environments. This occurred during my high school years, when I provided services as a hospital volunteer.

The Teapot

A person's soul is like water
in a teapot set upon a flame.
At first, it starts out
unperturbed and tame.
Then slowly possessed
by the penetrating heat
it boils in outbreaks of rage.
Then the heat is reduced
and the water begins to cool.
Eventually evaporating,
it leaves the pot cold and dry,
a useless tool.

— *Damon T. Arnold, MD*

This poem bothered me for some time. It was not only a bleak picture of where people had ended up in a final phase of their life on Earth but also an acknowledgment of the travesty that society supports the existence of such an outcome. It became apparent that an alternative view of life must be possible. The second poem has to do with the revelation that this was not an inevitable, predestined location for the seniors within our society.

One day, after working long hours practicing medicine, I took a walk on a colorful autumn day through a predominantly Asian community in Chicago. I walked by ornate restaurants and beautiful artwork, lanterns, and wooden carvings. I was deeply impressed by the truly beautiful people that dwelled in this community. I noticed children walking with their grandparents upon a cobblestone pathway down the street in a quiescent park.

It was then that I decided to walk into the park, as I was feeling tired and in need of some rest. Initially I felt that I could just benefit from some stress reduction by taking a walk. But by stopping to take this walk through the park, I gained a great deal more.

I saw senior citizens standing in a formation under the overarching branches of a revered, centuries-old oak tree. They moved silently and slowly through the graceful movements of a Tai Chi exercise. The younger members of their community stood watching with pride and awe at the level of sophistication and self-mastery their seniors had achieved over the course of their lifetimes. I later found out that this was a daily routine for them. They made it a functional part of their life course.

This experience allowed me to write this next poem, which attempted to capture the significance of this moment for me. I hope that this poem imparts a view of life that is useful for you as well. We must respect and cherish the positive contributions and accomplishments that others make throughout their lifetimes.

Falling Autumn Leaves

Transitory images spiraling above the planes
Within the wooden deep
Softly vibrated in the gentle breeze of forgetfulness
Being unbound from earthly concerns
To peer across the endless universal sea.
Bound by images of eternal youth rings
Glowing brightly within them
No dirge could pierce the silence and splendor
Of this flowing harmonious dance
Of universal oneness
Experienced by these autumn leaves falling.
For in their last earthly glimpses they view eternal life
Perfection and infinity lying before them
Which are held within their delicate hands.

— *Damon T. Arnold, MD*

The Tai Chi artists swirled, as did the leaves within the poem. During this experience, I realized that people can actually take charge of their personal lives and health outcomes. It is possible to have a life span filled with positivity and enjoyment that flowers into the perfection of one's sense of being and purpose throughout a lifetime. Once again, you hold the keys in your very hand for good or bad health outcomes and how you view life. Make sure to choose the keys that give you the best outcome possible.

Conflict Resolution and the Importance of Self-Control

I will begin by presenting a memory tool I devised to order my approach and response to situations involving interpersonal conflict. I have found that we live within a very complex societal web.

Within this realm, miscommunication and misinterpretation can predominate in instances of encountering interpersonal conflict. As a result, I have developed a simple memory tool that I use to gauge and respond to circumstances requiring conflict resolution.

When I was a child, I used to go to the beach at Coney Island in New York City with my brother and our friends with great enthusiasm, energy, and a crusading spirit of exploration. We used to search for seashells and swim along the sandy shores of the Atlantic Ocean. It was there that I was first introduced to the term *clam'n*, which describes the process of hunting for clams prior to a fish fry. At that point in life, I was revolted by the very thought of even contemplating putting one of those things in my mouth. Now I enjoy clam chowder with a sense of zeal. But the term *CLAM'N* also contains the letters associated with the various forms of conflict resolution.

Each letter represents the first letter in a term for a form of conflict resolution. They are arranged in order from the most restrictive and violent to the least restrictive and most peaceable form of communication in conflict resolution. I use this scale as a sort of barometer to gauge the level of conflict I am witnessing among the parties involved in a conflict. I use this at the meetings I attend as well, to obtain a sense of how the group members work together and whether they are likely to succeed.

These letters stand for **C**oercion, **L**itigation, **A**rbitration, **M**ediation, and **N**egotiation. Again, they are arranged in order from the highest to the lowest level of confrontational conflict. To clarify their intended uses, first I will define each of these approaches. Then I will discuss their roles in avoiding conflict escalations during the process of conflict resolution.

Coercion conveys the intent to dominate by force, as in a warlike way. It is a 'take no prisoners' stand that leaves many battle casualties and is all too often the entry point for disputes or disagreements. In these situations, I have witnessed that very rarely is the level of animus that arises actually tied to the actual problem or issue at hand.

Additionally, the 'enemy combatants' are rarely thinking with reason. Rather, they are reacting with emotions. In essence, they have blown past all the rational conflict-resolution levels that could have been utilized: negotiation, mediation, arbitration, and even litigation. They also are left with the negative consequences of this more violent approach.

Litigation involves a legal contest of sorts that is guided by a judicial process. This often involves civil misbehavior or criminal acts on the parts of the presenting parties. This is when the process is so out of control that the parties have to be told what to do to resolve the conflict. Essentially, no matter the reasons they have not been able to resolve their problems, they require legal intervention for an externally derived and binding solution.

Arbitration involves the use of an outside party that listens to the parties involved. This outside party resolves the dispute with decisions that are binding on the parties involved. This is a step down from litigation and is without the costs and formality of a legal proceeding. Yet the third party decision is binding and final.

Mediation involves the use of an outside party that helps the parties involved in a conflict to decide or settle upon a mutually agreed-upon resolution. The mediator guides the parties through the minefields of the conflict-resolution process. This helps the parties to meet under better circumstances and terms, enabling them to reach a shared resolution acceptable to each party involved. The final decision arises from the parties in conflict, and it is mutually binding.

Negotiation occurs when people confer on a rational basis with each other to reach a conflict resolution agreement. This is accomplished without outside intervention. Often I have found that this arena provides fertile ground for the exploration of potential commonalities and synergisms. These are often obscured by the presence of an 'individualistic' or 'silo-focused' viewpoint. The existence of such a silo focus is often enmeshed within and supported by an egocentric, emotionally immature, and explosive backdrop.

In approaching a conflict, there should always be an attempt to proceed under the lowest level of conflict resolution possible and practicable, which prevents further escalation. Despite the fact that many employees work together for long hours, little time if any is spent on addressing interpersonal communication.

Many times there is a failure to recognize the underlying problems spurring a more adversarial approach by the parties involved in the conflict-resolution process. It may be necessary to address other issues separately and to make known their distinction from the problem at hand.

I felt it was important to review here some of the stumbling blocks that prevent teamwork, progress, and ultimate goal attainments. I also noted in the title of this section the need for self-control.

One must also look at the surrounding social circumstances when negotiating with persons about the provision of an intervention service. The community members may have 'heard that tune before' and were disappointed at the final outcome of a proposed intervention strategy in the past. They may note that either it was never correctly implemented or it did not address their envisioned needs.

Denial is part of our defensive mechanism pool and shields us from confronting a seemingly insurmountable and emotionally based fact or situation. Elizabeth Kubler-Ross, MD, noted this in her work on the stages of death and dying.[3]

The tendencies toward denial along with situational adaptability can combine to shield us from the reality of the situation at hand. There is also much recent discussion on the link between inner-city social conditions and the risk for the development of post-traumatic stress disorder (PTSD). Carl Bell, MD, has put forth brilliant theories on the development of community resiliency skills that protect inner-city communities against the effects of negative factors encountered there.[4] His works are truly worth reading in detail. Such resiliency factors are extremely important to understand in approaching the provision of any intervention services to a community in need of them.

I started this book with a focus on intervention. I attempted to clearly state some of the principles and theories that I have found important so that whether you are a community member or interventionist you could benefit from them. There are many other references you can gain valuable viewpoints, information, and tools from. I have listed some further resources in the materials at the end of this book.

I will turn next to a discussion of the environment of the community. It is essential to understand the community infrastructure and the agents that we attempt to combat in an effort to prevent and reduce the consequences of morbidities and premature mortalities.

To accomplish this, in *Part 2* of this book, I will discuss several concepts regarding the environment in which we live. This will include several new views about the world in which we live and some considerations potential interventionists may wish to consider. The viewpoints I have constructed hopefully will aid you and provide thought for further elucidation of their validity and, most importantly, their relevance to the communities you serve.

---

[3]   Elizabeth Kubler-Ross, MD, *On Death and Dying* (Florence, Ky.: Routledge, 1969).

[4]   Carl Bell, MD, "Social and Emotional Costs of Learning Disabilities," *Perspective* 165 (2008): 174-75.

PART 2

Theories Concerning the Environment

Chapter 4

Words of Caution for Potential Interventionists

Interventionists must learn to understand the needs of those within the community being served. There are some words of caution as one makes an attempt to provide solutions to the perceived problems of people within a community. As a community interventionist, you must make a concerted effort to understand the viewpoints of those within the community. This involves the development of a capacity for understanding reality through the eyes of those you are attempting to help. This goes beyond a simple sense of empathy for those affected. It requires a full appreciation of what someone else desires, actually needs, and experiences as his or her unique reality. An important realization is that the process of intervention begins within you. However, this ultimately must be judged by the degree of conformity the outcome has with the community members' views on what constitutes success.

Discerning Wisdom from Dogma

Frankly, many times I am dissatisfied with the dogmatic jargon arising within both the academic and medical arenas. When I was in training, there were those seated upon the throne of status-quo mediocrity. They would, in an almost parrot-like way, recite scientific facts mixed with an arsenal of unscientific dogma, proudly parading it as superior thinking. This dogma was sometimes of a scientific nature, such as performing hysterectomies—many of which were later found to be unnecessary. Dogma often thrives within an environment of status-quo mediocrity, which blindly resists innovation attempts directed at the scientific validation of changes that are beneficial to society. But the most glaring and destructive of these was the blatant disregard for and artificially contrived views of the community being serviced.

I will now discuss the theoretical underpinnings of a more rational and logical approach to community engagement. As with any new idea, skeptics with little vision or insight will abound. Take, for example, the early astronomers or chemists that were ostracized or literally beheaded. They were attacked by skeptics because their ideas were visionary and often diametrically opposed to and in conflict with the prevailing viewpoints, beliefs, and dogmas of the culture in which they tried to introduce them.

The points of view of these innovators and scientists were valid as supported by the evolving scientific method. However, they could not withstand the often violent resistance offered by the collective consciousness of those in political power that reacted to these new ideas.

The rulers of the societies in which they attempted to insert these new ideas flatly rejected the visionaries' views. These rulers were threatened by what they could not comprehend or control.

Many of the visionaries were treated as heretics and sorcerers. This was because of the wide gap between their level of thinking and understanding and that of those that opposed their views—to whom they appeared to be practicing witchcraft, heresy, or magic. Further, the rulers mistakenly and arrogantly believed they knew everything and had all the answers required. But, as I noted earlier, they were not aware that a different approach to the question at hand was even possible of being entertained, because of their lack of vision and self-imposed blindness. They were largely blinded by traditional dogmatic thinking with the added touch of their arrogance. The educational process for those who are not able to comprehend new concepts can be daunting and costly both in time and resources. Such persons still exist in modern society.

These individuals may also impart a negative effect by contaminating the process for healing within a community by offering 'solutions' cloaked in archaic and prejudicial beliefs and practices. Their logic is warped by these destructive viewpoints, which concern the very community members they say they wish to help. These attempts then masquerade as 'solutions' to community-based problems, which subsequently fail. This further erodes community trust in the overall process of not only this intervention but also any subsequent interventions. For those who are of this type, it is better for you to work on your 'self' first. Once this is accomplished, you can then address the problems confronting the community members you are attempting to help.

False 'solutions' become superimposed upon, and are often detrimental to, the social identities of the community members themselves. How such an unethical and immoral practice persists to this day escapes any rational explanation. Therefore, an assessment of how and whether a contemplated intervention does or does not fit in with the views of community members is essential—before its implementation.

It is imperative for all partners involved to focus on the same goals, objectives, and metric tools with respect to the intended intervention. This is essential for ensuring that the collaborative efforts and synergisms arising from such a partnership group are mutually acceptable, coordinated, and ultimately effective. It was essential for me to emphasize the reality and existence of the observations I have encountered over the years. Hiding behind the cloaks of denial and falsehoods will hinder any further steps toward true progress in healing within communities and our nation as a whole. While participating in various community interventions in the past, I found several problems with intervention attempts. It was apparent that inadequate dialogue existed for the validation or modification of the effectiveness of the attempted community interventions. They were never field tested for situational and contextual effectiveness, based upon appropriate community member feedback.

This lack of communication and community engagement has resulted in a less-than-progressive approach to resolving the issues surrounding individual and community health concerns. In fact, it has alienated many of the community members from efforts at future care.

This disregard for true dialogue, along with the falsely constructed cultural views, was largely created by people who were not a part of the community being serviced. In fact, most often there was very little, if any, input sought from the community members in the attempt to solve the problems they confronted as a community. In addition, the interventionists blatantly rejected the creation of new ideas or view—that is, those that did not originate with them or their like-minded colleagues.

They were actually often a hindrance to true scientific discovery, community engagement, and progress. Many of them frankly rejected the integration of medicine with information technology, business theory, behavioral sciences, marketing, universal health coverage, complementary forms of health practice, and many other areas of organized community activity. We are now facing many of the social consequences of such poor decisions.

Currently these areas are the "hot topics" being brought forward by the very ones that rejected their relevance previously. Further, their exploration of the communities they serviced stopped at the front doors of the academic or medical service establishments they worked in. These so called 'ivory towers' did provide some of the greatest medical discoveries in modern times for treatment. However, little, if anything, was actually done to truly engage the community members being serviced. And no significant effort was made to correct infrastructure problems or to prevent the occurrence of diseases within the conceptual settings of serviced communities.

Recipients of intervention services must be intimately involved in this process for it to succeed. The views of community members must be explored and an explanation of the intended intervention provided. Many of the community members' views have been largely shaped by the imposition by those in power of negative stereotypes and misrepresentations of the community members themselves. These are American citizens—whether in the inner city or on a farm—and should be respected as such.

The Fallacies of Logic

Fallacies of logic are faulty, illogical assertions that lead to invalid and erroneous conclusions. I have noticed that when people are involved in problem-resolution discussions, they often rely on poorly constructed and faulty statements and assertions. In fact, they attempt to assert them as valid logical conclusions. I will start with definitions of the terms *argument* and *logic* as they appear in the *Merriam Webster's Collegiate Dictionary*, tenth edition. I will then present many of the fallacies of logic, with examples, which mislead by giving an erroneous appearance of treading upon the well-reasoned path of logic.

> **Argument**: [noun; Latin—'argumentum', 'arguer'—to make clear] A discussion in which disagreement is expressed: debate. A quarrel or a reason or matter for dispute or contention. A course of reasoning aimed at demonstrating the 'truth' or 'falsehood' of something. A fact or statement offered as proof or evidence. It is a summary of the plot or subject of a literary work. The minor premise is a syllogism. In math: the independent variable of a function or the amplitude of a complex number.

> **Logic**: [noun; ME *logic*, Fr. MF *logique*, . . . of reason] 1 a (1): a science that deals with the principles and criteria of validity of inference and demonstration: the science of the formal principles of reasoning . . .

What follows is the description of 13 fallacies of logic. They can be reviewed here. An attempt should be made to remember and use them when listening to or participating in a discussion or argument. They can be remembered by a mnemonic I crafted: *FAR EAST PEACE B.* The components are listed below in this order.

1. The *false analogy* assumes that because things are similar in some ways, they are in all ways. For example, the dog has four legs

55

and so does the table. Since the dog can run down the road, so can the table.

2. An *argumentum ad hominem* appeals to a person's biases and emotions rather than to logic or reason. For example, a person may assert, knowing that the individual he or she is talking to is hungry, "The meal must taste good. Just take a look at it. Don't you agree?" This is asserted to convince someone, despite never actually tasting the meal, by appealing to that person's sense of hunger and reasoned input.

3. The *red herring* changes the subject to distract the audience of listeners from the true issue at hand. "That athlete beat everyone in the marathon, but just look at how bad his shoes are."

4. The use of *equivocation* is an attempt to shift the meaning of a key word. This occurs through the use of vague, ambiguous, or misleading language. "This product has all-natural ingredients" gives one the feeling that the product must be good for one's health—despite containing 'all natural' high-fructose corn syrup that can lead to obesity, morbidity, and a premature death.

5. An *argumentum ad ignorantum* occurs when someone asserts that something is true because it cannot be proven to be false. I could note that the pyramids were constructed with the guidance of alien life forms. This statement might hold if it had to rely on our being transported in time to support or disprove it, no matter how unlikely my assertion may be. This can also establish the basis for myths and dogmatic beliefs that persist for generations.

6. *Skewing the sample* results when one shifts the distribution of a population from one to another. This can occur when one attempts to generalize a statement. For example, one may note that all aircraft with wings have an ability to glide to the ground should the engines suddenly stall. However, helicopters are also called rotary wing aircraft and cannot glide should the engine stall.

7. An *argument tu quoque* occurs when a person is accused of not upholding the position for which he or she is advocating. An example is when someone who is overweight is advocating for good nutrition or dieting. The fact that the person is overweight does not negate the fact that what he or she is saying is valid.

8. A *post hoc* error in logic arises when one establishes an improper link between cause and effect. 'The reason that it rained is because I left my car windows down.'

9. The *either-or fallacy* involves treating a complex issue as though it were simple to solve. "All you need is a rocket attached to a cabin to land on the moon."

10. An *argument ad populum* involves an appeal to the prejudices of the audience. "We should go to war with them because everybody knows they hate us all!"

11. A *consensus gentium* argument involves trying to establish that something is true because "everyone" thinks so. "Everyone knows that you cannot make a living by becoming an artist, so why try?" That is, despite the fact that living affluent artists exist.

12. An *evasion of the issue* occurs when a person evades focusing on and dealing directly with the issue at hand. "Despite there being a fire in the house, we need to focus on finishing the planting of seeds in the garden."

13. *Begging the question* involves stating a debatable premise as if it were valid. "That was the best movie ever made!"

Enter the New Approaches

Due to the contributions of some truly dedicated and community-centered practitioners, interventionists in general began to talk of such things as cultural and linguistic competency as well as community partnerships. Although unable to locate their exact origin or authors,

I have run across these maxims during my studies and practice, which I feel are words to the wise.

"All models are wrong—but, some are useful."

"In God we trust. All others bring data."

"Fear is bad counsel."

It must be kept in mind that there are numerous models and theories within the academic, medical, and community settings. These interventions can be scientific, quasi-scientific, or observational in nature. There are many good scientific tools for conceptualizing intervention strategies. However, despite having a valid scientific basis, some models can be operationally invalid and even harmful. From a community point of view, both positive and negative concepts may be either acceptable or unacceptable, depending on the method utilized to introduce them. Obviously, the invalid or harmful ones should be weeded out.

Depending upon how they are perceived and valued by the community, these invalid or harmful interventions may take root and thrive. This then perpetuates harm and possibly results in an established dogmatic practice that may be very difficult to eradicate. However, it may also be as simple as educating community members about the potential harmful outcome should they use the invalid or harmful intervention.

Likewise, if you are able to discern a highly effective intervention, there may be no need to 'reinvent the wheel,' which tends to waste valuable amounts of your, and others, time, energy, and resources. However, you will have to develop an approach to gain the acceptance and buy-in of community members for the planned intervention to be successful.

The Exercise

As a senior medicine resident and attending physician, I would send my assigned medical students and medicine residents through an exercise.

I would pick a case that was difficult to diagnose and then have them see the patient. The one rule was that they were not allowed to look into the patient's chart or ask any of the other medical professionals about the patient's diagnosis. The following is what happened in one particular case.

> The case involved the presence of a skin lesion on a woman who had recently immigrated to the United States from the Middle East and who was not particularly talkative. I sent an internal medicine resident in to see her and told him to meet me in the cafeteria in an hour, where I would be awaiting his diagnosis. After a period of time he arrived, frantically ready to report his guess at the diagnosis.
>
> However, at that point I gave him some money and told him to get the healthiest thing he could find to eat and to make sure to get some water. He shortly returned with a tray and placed it in front of me. I then asked him what his diagnosis was for the lady he examined.
>
> He began by stating that the lesion appeared to be a bacterial infection of the skin. I noted that it could have been, but that it was not. I then opened and raised a newspaper between us and began to read it.
>
> The medicine resident went on to note that it could be a skin lesion caused by a virus. I told him it could have been, but it was not. Then he noted that it could be skin cancer. Again, I told him it was not. He then seemed uncomfortable with the newspaper between us and moved his chair as if to communicate directly with me. Then he asked me, *"Why are you not paying attention and listening to me?"* At that point, I put the newspaper down.
>
> I explained that when I sent him into the room to examine the lady with the skin lesion, he failed to do several things. The first was to realize that you largely see what you read. I explained that he was not going to reinvent the field of medicine when he walked into the room. We are largely parrots in this world, simply repeating what we have heard repeatedly before. Much of what we do and say in medicine is built upon our reliance on the works of millions of

people who contributed to the field over thousands of years before our entrance into it.

This goes back to ancient times to include all world cultures. Occasionally, there are sparks of true genius that occur, but generally people operate by routine protocols. They proceed in a parrot-like fashion to act on amassed knowledge gained from didactic and experiential learning or training.

The actual diagnosis was blastomycosis of the skin, a relatively rare fungal skin infection to encounter in our hospital at that time. He did not recognize it, as he had not read about or seen it before. I explained to him that if someone were to grow up around and only be exposed to the presence of oak trees, then every tree they saw in the forest would appear to be an oak tree. There is no room for variation or imagination, as the person has never been exposed to or considered the existence of another type of tree, such as a pine tree.

This is true for everything we experience. If the environment you are constantly exposed to is a food desert, you will think in terms of the unhealthy foods present there if you have never seen healthier foods. If you experience hunger, you will seek these unhealthy foods out in an attempt to satisfy your hunger. However, this falls very far from the goal of meeting your actual nutritional needs and a healthy lifestyle. Absent being educated about or having actual exposure to an environment that offers healthy alternatives, no other perceived choices exist for you other than the unhealthy foods.

I went on to explain that the lady knew her diagnosis. Although she was a bit reserved with respect to speaking to strangers, she would have told him the diagnosis if he had simply asked her. You see, I had instructed him not to talk to other health professionals, but I never told him not to talk to the patient. His sole focus on and persistence in trying to find an answer to this diagnostic puzzle caused him to lose sight of the partnership with the person he was trying to assist. In essence he had established a wall, much like I had done with the newspaper locking him out. This engagement with her was vitally important in providing any form of assistance to her.

In addition, it was never his diagnosis alone, as he had entered a partnership with a human being who needed his help and assistance with their health status. The diagnosis of most community-based problems involves an exchange of hot air between the interventionist and the person requiring assistance—that is, a dialogue with effective communication occurring.

I then told him to eat the meal and drink the water. He had a perplexed look. He noted that he had bought the food for me with my money. I told him that the food and water were for him.

I wanted him to learn three things from this meal, which I explained to him. First, although I had indicated that he should buy the meal, I never indicated the meal was intended for me or that I would ultimately accept it from him. Second, in order to take care of others, you must also learn to take care of yourself. The meal also had to be a healthy one, for if you preach health, you must also practice it. Third, I saw that he was hungry as well and decided to perform an act of compassion myself. Do not pass this opportunity up when working with clients or colleagues.

One can have an abundance of energy and passion in what one does but completely miss the mark. Adolf Hitler had passion but brought a great deal of pain, suffering, and premeditated murders into the world. His passion was tied to an evil intent that was blind to morality and ethical behavior. In short, your passion must be bound to compassion for all those you encounter to have a positive effect. I truly feel that the ability to combine passion with compassion is the highest form of human development. Reaching the pinnacle of human development involves successfully blending the highest ideals of emotional, cognitive, and spiritual development with compassion and then putting them into action.

In the next chapter I discuss a conceptual view I created to unify the eastern and western concepts and theories of scientific thought.

Chapter 5

The Eastern-Western Bridge

At first glance, the paradigms of Eastern and Western science appear to be distinctly different conceptual frameworks. However, they both have a common origin in the attempt to explain occurrences within the natural environment. Each is an attempt to explain energy-matter relationships that constantly surround and indeed comprise us all. In this chapter, I will define these paradigms and blend them into a universal conceptual model.

Eastern Inductive and Western Deductive Reasoning

I have created an "energy-matter spectrum" concept. This concept goes beyond the traditional perspective of an electromagnetic spectrum. It represents a unified theory inclusive of all energy-matter relationships in existence. It also integrates the concepts of Eastern and Western scientific viewpoints. This spectrum extends from light wave and particle physics theory to the biological kingdoms containing the food chains. It includes all natural and man-made energy-matter relationships currently in existence.

Humans are probably at the top of this list evolutionarily. I say 'probably' at the top because of the destructive interactions humans have had with the environment over the course of time. Also, as people view Eastern and Western medicine from their Western or Eastern viewpoints, they often place one of them on a pedestal while the other is looked down upon with disdain. The truth is that both have their applications and drawbacks. They both are extremely valuable to us all. They require adept practitioners who have dedicated themselves to practice with a high degree of competence and compassion.

All of the buildings and inventions that surround us are just the result of the application of our intellect in the construction of what we call reality. We developed physically to interact and deal with our environment. Then we began to contemplate the creation of tools for arranging and constructing the myriad human artifacts that surround us. This is a miraculous achievement that has landed a man on the surface of the Earth's moon and spacecraft on the planet Mars. These efforts have largely relied upon cognitive reasoning and a scientific approach toward interaction with the environment. The use of both inductive and deductive reasoning underlie the scientific process.

The epitome of deductive reasoning is categorical syllogism: premise—premise—conclusion. For example, all cars have four wheels; there is a car down the street; therefore the car must have four wheels. One moves from the general to the specific. This is in contradistinction to inductive reasoning, in which one goes from the specific to the general.

The epitome of inductive reasoning is the analogy. For example, you may hold a single grain of sand in your hand and notice that it feels coarse. If you were then to view a beach covered with sand, you would generalize your experience based on a single grain of sand. You would reach the conclusion that the vast accumulations of sand grains before you would all be coarse were you to touch them. A generalized pattern emerges in this way, which is a key concept in Eastern scientific thought.

Western science attempts to dissect and fragment parts while labeling and categorizing them, sometimes ignoring their cohesion and interconnectedness. Observation and experimentation devoid of human emotion, and to some degree experiential input, have been the hallmarks of this approach. As a result, Western science has at times departed from a connection with our emotional and spiritual development, even putting their very existences into question. This occurs as we view human emotions and spirituality through the filter of this isolated and detached scientific lens. However, this approach also has several strengths, and it has led to many scientific breakthroughs throughout recorded history, even in its earlier and less formalized approaches.

Both the Eastern and the Western approaches have their strengths and drawbacks. They are merely two different conceptual approaches to the same energy-matter relationships that surround us all. Exactly how many other conceptual viewpoints and reasoning patterns are truly possible remain to be discovered.

Whether one agrees with the Western or Eastern viewpoint, it should be recognized that each has arrived at valid, time-proven approaches and results. They both have brought into fruition undeniable and valid approaches to the prevention and treatment of injury, illness, and disease.

The Eastern-Western Bridge

I have converted the limited, traditional Western-based electromagnetic spectrum into a more expansive *energy-matter spectrum*. This includes Eastern scientific approaches as well. I have often commented to my public health and medical staffs over the years that *"the energy matter spectrum extends from particle physics to the food chain, and we deal with every aspect of it in our work."*

The Eastern approach relies upon the interrelationship of arrayed points in space that form characteristic relationships, arrangements, and patterns. In applying the energy-matter spectrum concept to the Eastern viewpoint, I equate yang (pronounced *young*) with the Western concept of *energy* and yin with the Western concept of *matter*.

Yang embodies the Western concept of energy, although it is quite a bit more expansive than the Western correlate. The Eastern concept can be envisioned as a man running on a hot, sun-drenched beach with his arms and hands outstretched and expansive clouds far above. Water is evaporating as waves spread across the sand. Everything is bright, high energy, and expansive. This is the bright side of the mountain.

The Eastern concept of the Western-based concept of mass is yin. This can be visualized as a pregnant woman in a cold, dark cave. Further, the moon is out and a mixture of snow and rain fall upon the darkened trees sprouting up from the ground outside the cave. Everything is dark, low energy, and contracting. Note that this embodies the acts of matter creation as well as the perpetuation of life forms. This is the dark side of the mountain.

It should be noted that both yang (energy) and yin (matter) are always present in varying amounts in both our surrounding environment and within our very own bodies. For example, the evaporation of sweat cools the body of a man on a beach, preventing his death from heat exhaustion. The pregnant woman in the cave shivers to warm her body, preventing her death by hypothermia.

The relationship of yang (lightness) and yin (darkness) is represented in the Eastern symbol of the Tai Ji and can be extended to Western concepts of energy-matter relationships as described in Figure 1.

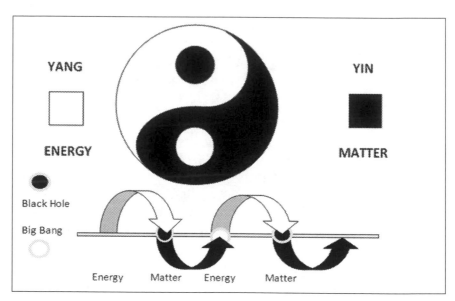

Figure 1. Tai Ji transformed into an energy-matter sine wave (low point on sine wave is matter and high point is energy)

In Figure 1 the black color moving in a downward motion within the circle represents both the formation of matter itself and the solidification of the earth (order). The white color represents an upward movement toward the formation of energy (disorder).

However, each of these contains a circle bearing the opposite color within it. Therefore, matter does not exist without energy in any meaningful way. Energy does not exist without matter in any meaningful way. I speculate that these circles represent the resistance against the total transformation of accumulated energy into pure energy and accumulated matter into pure matter. Both of these states need to be present in a balanced relationship and would have little if any meaning without the presence of the other. From an astronomical viewpoint, perhaps the dark circle represents a black hole in the midst of a field of high-energy input, while the white circle represents a big bang in the midst of a dense-matter field input.

Actually, for mass or energy to have any real meaning, there must be the representation of mass in energy and energy in mass. For example, the bright energy of a standard light bulb must contain the mass of a filament and thin, solid glass globe to work. Likewise, the bulky mass of a truck must be associated with energy not only to provide movement but also just to hold it together as a solid object.

This energy–matter spectrum is a bridge that can be utilized for the further exploration, elucidation, and potential integration of Eastern and Western theoretical viewpoints. In fact, what is considered to be Western scientific thought actually began in Eastern cultures. It is interesting that both 'Western' and 'Eastern' scientific thought actually had their origins in the East.

Energy-matter relationships may also be viewed as the basis for the development of susceptibility to—or an innate resiliency against—a negative or a positive consequence that arises within a community. If we apply this view to order and disorder, we have their correlates of black (matter/yin) and white (energy/yang), respectively. The relative balance between these two states—matter and energy—would be present within the environment. However, a tendency toward stability or instability is represented by the circles in Figure 1 as black or white, respectively. Both stability (order) and instability (disorder) are necessary for change to occur, and neither should be looked upon as being undesirable in and of itself. Both are necessary for adaptability and survival.

When the stability or instability leads to a change with a higher relative risk for a negative social consequence, we set the stage for negative social disruptions and the ensuing consequences of poor health. With the occurrence of a change in a negative direction and the resultant crystallization of a negative consequence, impacted community members experience an increase in morbidity and premature mortality.

It may be apparent that a grocery store in a food desert should be demolished. It is in gross disrepair and sells products that are harmful to community members. However, making a change requires a certain level of instability. The removal of this establishment requires the instability created by a construction wrecking crew. It would be a positive and progressive move for the community members if this dysfunctional business with its negative community impact were removed. It must, however, be replaced with an establishment that provides healthy, nutritional alternatives within this food desert community.

This change will provide a progressive, positive impact within the community environment. However, a movement toward the demolition of an old building to be replaced by another high-calorie, fast-food establishment would be associated with the continuation of negative and destructive social consequences. Therefore, the ability to manipulate the environment through efforts directed at stabilization or destabilization can each be constructive or destructive in its effects with respect to realized good health outcomes.

The Elements of Nature

You may be familiar with another viewpoint from Eastern philosophy. This involves the concept of the elements of nature: earth, water, fire, metal, and wood. After considering these elements for some time and their interrelationships, I conjectured that what they actually may represent is an ancient technological advancement.

They appeared to me to be related in the following way:

I visualized a metallic stand holding a metallic cup on an earthen floor. A wood pile on the earth was on fire beneath the metallic cup, which contained boiling water generating steam. This may have been the advent of a more sophisticated form of cooking, but I could not easily dismiss the image of a relationship that contained all the elements. They were interacting, and there was a continuous transformation occurring. Further, the evaporated water could no longer be visualized and appeared to enter a spiritual world, as it could no longer be seen by the observer. This would then join the clouds to return later as rain falling upon the earth to nourish the wooden trees. And the cycle would repeat itself. The art of cooking food and boiling water represented a tremendous technological breakthrough for the health and wellness of human civilization. If I am correct, it is no wonder that these essential elements gained such symbolic prominence in the Eastern cultural experience.

However, all paradigms have their dogmatic shortcomings. We must continually strive to understand our relative position within the universal environment, beginning within ourselves. One of the essential qualities of these energy-matter relationships is the ability to change and adapt. Likewise, we must be able to change our emotional and mental views—so as not to be stagnated by identification with a behavioral or thought pattern that causes us to experience increased morbidity and possibly a premature death. Change your behavior and make a personal investment in solving your particular personal and social problems, which we all bare. Flexibility allows for adaptability in nature, life, and scholarship. We must remember what we are essentially doing is asking people to attempt to change their behaviors with an intervention plan. We must be willing to do the same.

There are several Eastern health practices in existence. There is a basic definition of several arts listed in the glossary section of this book. I have written a book, *The Silent Gray Serpent,* which is soon to be released, that presents a much more detailed and thorough discussion of these practices.

In the next chapter, I provide a basic discussion of the environmental link to individual and community health. The environment is gaining increasing attention as the links between disease and environmental infrastructure problems and contamination become more established. For instance, asthma and air pollution have strongly established environmental linkages. These concerns will grow exponentially in the years to come as the deleterious environmental impact of humankind continues in a largely unabated fashion. Currently, global security and survival rests in the hands of the human race. Hopefully, the correct decisions will be made.

Chapter 6

The Environmental Link to Your Health

Links between environmental agents and the health consequences of pain, suffering, and premature death are continually being established. People are exposed to environmental agents that originate at every point within the energy-matter spectrum. This includes such environmental agents as radon in our basements, caustic cleaning chemicals under our sinks, lead or asbestos on or in walls, and bacteria and viruses in the kitchen and bathroom. Various insects carrying infectious diseases and multiple species of spiders are the inhabitants of the average home. These agents interact and leave humanity with the dilemma of how to deal with the impacts they create.

Toxins, Toxins Everywhere

We confront and are exposed to many of these environmental agents and toxins on a continuous basis. They are present at work, in the community, and at home. These exposures occur over various periods and in various types and degrees of exposure. What I propose is that any potential agent we encounter be placed in sequence along an energy-matter spectrum, (Figure 2). Albert Einstein's equation, $E = mc^2$, can be rearranged to form the energy-matter spectrum continuum I am speaking of.

Einstein's equation, involving the relationships between

mass (m), energy (E), and the speed of light squared (c^2), which can be expressed as

$$E = mc^2$$

On paper, this can be rearranged to form

$$E/c^2 \text{ (Energy)} = M \text{ (Matter)}$$

Figure 2. Einstein's equation

This is the basis of the energy-matter spectrum that extends through a spectrum of increasing complexity from pure energy to dense, complex matter. As one progresses through this spectrum, an individual agent's composition becomes a more complex energy-matter relationship. That is, it progresses sequentially through light, energy waves, subatomic particles, atoms, chemicals, biochemicals, prions, viruses, bacteria, and on to the life forms within the five biological kingdoms. The biological component of this spectrum also includes the food chains that meet our nutritional needs. Any of these levels can be a source of agents that are toxic to human life.

Each organism contains within, a combination of the various energy-matter states and relationships that exist within the surrounding natural energy-matter spectrum. For example, the human body contains nerve cells with electrical currents, lungs with gases, vessels with fluids, soft tissues, and solid bone.

A New View of the Public Health Spectrum of Responsibility

From a historical perspective, infectious diseases have become the focal point of what public health is and does. However, the overall energy-matter spectrum demonstrates a more accurate and expansive view of the public health domain in modern times.

In an incredibly complex society, public health covers issues concerning nuclear and other forms of energy, chemical exposures, viruses, bacteria, the human genome, and food safety and nutritional concerns. Agents can act within various environments and periods of time to result in pain, suffering, and a premature death. Likewise, work, community, and home environments are inextricably linked to your health. Each of the points falling along the spectrum can be viewed as a specific agent with the potential for doing harm, whether in the home, work, or community environments.

Exposure to too much sunlight can cause skin cancer. Drinking too much water can cause water intoxication. Exposure to lead in paint chips can cause lead poisoning. Viruses or bacteria can cause infections. Overeating food can cause obesity and chronic disease. Drinking alcohol during pregnancy can lead to fetal alcohol spectrum disorders in the unborn child. There is also speculation that the ingestion of certain foods by pregnant women may lead to the development of childhood allergies in their children.

What matters are the quality, concentration, and quantity of an agent or substance and the degree of bodily exposure over a given time period. You can swallow, inhale, or have your skin covered with an agent or toxin. The intensity of exposure can vary in the case of multiple, recurrent exposures. It is also possible to have an abnormal reaction to an agent or allergen, such as peanuts, pollen, or shellfish. Many disease states are made worse by exposure to environmental substances, such as cigarette smoke complicating or triggering an asthma attack.

In the modern world, we are inundated by environmental pollutants. The long-term effects of many of these agents, especially when present in various combinations, are unknown at this time. However, some agents are known to be directly related to chronic diseases and even cancer.

Much work needs to be done with respect to issues related to these agents. This requires the dedication of resources, research, and commitment. Most importantly, it requires both the recognition and a lack of denial about this problem's existence as a major societal problem that is intimately related to our health status outcomes.

Historically, we not only witnessed the appearance of toxic substances within our workplaces during the industrial age but also their extension into our community and home environments. Economically deprived communities are often the recipients of agents from industrial processes and consequences; these are found in proximity of community member's homes. This is due to several factors, including such issues as lower land costs and access to a cheaper labor force. There is also less ability among poor community members to mount a significant oppositional response to industry-based intrusions into their community settings. They are often not a part of the most privileged "Not In My Back Yard" (NIMBY) group that can fend off, to a much greater degree, the placement of pollution sources within their communities.

We are in a world where death by environmental suicide has been taking place. Global warming, coral reef depletion, toxic waste dump accumulations, wetland disappearance, and deforestation have accelerated over the past several decades. It is a well-known fact that the United States uses approximately 25 percent of the petroleum produced in the world, while representing only approximately 5 percent of the world's total population. However, industrialization is also increasing in an uncontrolled fashion in several developing countries at alarming rates.

We must confront and contend with these environmental mishaps and prevent their potential for inflicting human pain, suffering, and premature deaths, to which we are all susceptible. The point is that none of us can stand idly by and assume that environmental contamination does not apply to and will not affect us or our family members directly.

Injuries, whether accidental or intentional, are merely the results of energy-matter relationship interactions. An accidental car crash or a speeding bullet in an act of violence both represent energy-matter relationships that result in injury. Injuries are a leading cause of death, especially in younger individuals and the elderly.

In *Part 3* of this book, I will present my Theory of Social Disruption model in detail. The theory of social disruption model relies upon the energy-matter conceptual view explained above. Further, this model is intended to provide a conceptual framework for understanding and defining various community-based variables that affect health outcomes.

PART 3

The Community Social Disruption Model

The Raindrop

In the purest of clouds
A raindrop is born.
It is perplexed by the invisible winds
That change its form.
As it falls, a gaze reveals
That some raindrops fall
Through the multihued rainbow of dawn
While others pass through clouds dark and strange.
Finally hitting the concrete,
Missing the fine, trim lawn,
It intermingles with other raindrops fallen,
All becoming one entity,
And desperately tries to regain
Its lost identity.
This is the life of the city child
Who disappears into obscure regression,
Having been born into overwhelming,
Poverty and oppression.

— *Damon T. Arnold, MD*

Chapter 7

The Missing Line for Social Disruption

During my time as a medical care provider, the following issue became vividly apparent to me. When the provision of medical care is mixed with social justice and poverty issues, therapeutic approaches and interventions need to be drastically modified. There appeared to be an absence of connection to the realities of everyday community life.

Giving a patient a diagnosis without an effective treatment plan offers little in the way of help. In effect, this is analogous to telling a patient that they are about to drive off the edge of a cliff in a car that happens to be without brakes. In this way, the medical and social support systems fail to provide an intervention strategy and safety net as an effective response to the issues community members are encountering—that is, a way to prevent community members from succumbing to pain, suffering, and premature death.

This is particularly true if society supports, from a socioeconomic standpoint, continued production of, existence of, and exposure to risk factor agents. This may include the support of for-profit businesses that impart morbidity and premature mortality as a result of their business practices – that is, with no intended mechanisms to eliminate the resultant negative health outcomes. This is also often accompanied by the relative lack of cultural and linguistic competency on the part of the providers of such destructive services and products within at-risk communities. In fact, the vast majority of these business benefactors reside outside the impoverished and unstable community settings in which they establish their businesses.

COL. Damon T. Arnold, M.D., M.P.H.

As a resident physician at Cook County Hospital in Chicago, I was expected to record notes on a patient's medical history in his or her chart. There was also a required physical examination and ordering of relevant diagnostic tests. This sequence of events would allow us to arrive at one or more definitive diagnoses.

This information was essentially organized as sections of a patient history, an assessment, and a plan of care. It roughly corresponded to the patient's *subjective* complaint of symptoms, *objective* physical findings, an *assessment* of the person's over-all medical status, and a *plan* for further care (aka, 'SOAP' notes). The plan section included a treatment regimen, such as medication use, and further diagnostic studies or treatment interventions.

It became vividly clear early in my residency that the diagnostic and treatment lines in the chart should have been followed by what I call a social disruption line. Clearly, many times a diagnosis, such as Stage IV cancer, and its treatments should have been followed by a line denoting the stage or degree of social disruption—that is, the social conditions a patient was returning to when they went home. Many people were frankly returning to what I would call Stage IV social disruption. This social disruption line reflects the socioeconomic conditions that patients had to return to. The relative level of social disruption would dramatically affect the outcomes of the treatments and strategies we enacted to address their specific medical diagnoses.

To have a successful or better treatment outcome, they would ultimately have to independently deal with these various factors, often on their own. These community environments were often very poorly equipped with the level of support needed to meet a patient's needs. Medical staff members often said that a patient's social conditions were too complex and formidable to deal with. Yet, in virtually the same breath, they would note that they were going to take on curing cancer in that individual.

It was quite obvious that the social environment plays a major role in recovery and in adherence to medical treatment plans. For example, placing morbidly obese diabetic patients on a 1,200 calorie ADA diet before discharge without dietary counseling seemed absurd. From the hospital windows, I witnessed many of them head to eat at the nearest street vendor or fast-food establishment immediately upon discharge from the hospital and before leaving for home on the mass transit system.

The point is that it would not be long before they were once again out of balance—after having eaten over 2,000 calories just at the vendor's cart. I realized that this could result in subsequent hospital admissions for urgent care, if the person even chose to return to the hospital after a treatment failure. It could even result in the untimely death of the patient.

The Problem of Intervention Plans and Infrastructure Incompatibilities

I was puzzled by why we would hand out pictures of brightly colored food pyramids. I was already quite aware of food deserts' at the community level in the early 1980s in Chicago and while growing up in an impoverished community in Brooklyn, New York. Why would we give such a document out to people returning to a community that only had access to *"Potatoes in the form of 14 different flavors of potato chips, and tomatoes in the form of tomato ketchup,"* as noted by Congressman Bobby Rush, a US representative in Illinois's First Congressional District and member of the Congressional Black Caucus.

Perhaps on a subconscious level, these providers were attempting to treat their own inadequacies—that is, their inability to understand the basic principles and realities in operation in the community they were attempting to serve but had never visited.

Although only recently noted in the literature, food deserts have been in existence for many decades, if not hundreds of years, in disparately impacted communities worldwide. In fact, any major stadium, even if in an affluent area, is a form of food desert when one considers what is sold as food in these establishments. For example, only nachos and hot dogs may be available.

Consideration of the underlying stability of the critical infrastructure and key resource sectors within the community to which a patient is being discharged are vitally important to the success of any therapeutic regimen. This brings into focus the fact that several destructive forces are in operation within impacted communities. These forces should not be confused with the array of unhealthy options that exist, such as unhealthy foods and poor living conditions. In other words, the dilapidated surroundings within a blighted community are the result of an institutionalized pattern of societal forces that results in their emergence and their continued presence. Poor education and cultural brainwashing are simply not some form of *de novo* manifestation but rather result from intentional acts that orchestrate their occurrence.

Note that difficulty with transportation and a relative lack of mobility further exacerbate the social isolation experienced by members within these communities. The provision of inadequate transportation services is ultimately based upon poorly constructed and inadequate social and economic policies. Further, community targeting for the introduction of unhealthy products is inextricably linked to the appearance of chronic diseases with the associated consequences of pain, suffering, and premature deaths. The entry of unhealthy products into these communities is partly a manifestation of the free market system.

The Need for Policy Reform within the Built Environment

The inability of community members to make choices between healthy and unhealthy products is based on both socioeconomic and geopolitical grounds. This is largely due to the fact that healthy alternatives usually do not exist in a food desert and are difficult and relatively expensive to procure.

In fact, the absence of healthy alternatives has a great deal to do with how the geopolitical and social overtones that impact a 'food desert' community are structured. Affluent society members may in fact support such a construct if it is socially and economically beneficial to their interest. These factors make possible the emergence of 'invisible' subpopulations with a high degree of morbidity and premature mortality. It may seem easier for the general society to deny or destroy the credibility of these disparately impacted subpopulations than to resolve the social impacts the community members are experiencing. This is especially true if a profit motive is in operation for those who are more affluent.

After all, it takes energy and courage to recognize the true origin of these impacts. This often occurs only after one crosses the threshold of his or her personal discomfort, disgust, and outright contempt for those community members. They say there is no hope for these community members and that there is nothing that can be gained from this experience. "They will not buy healthy foods if we offered them anyway." Correct? Wrong! Some of the most powerful people in history have arisen within such social circumstances. Albert Einstein lived in poverty, was persecuted by the Nazi SS, and still became one of the greatest scientists of the twentieth century.

However, Einstein was still a great friend to Paul Robeson and served as the co-chair of the anti-lynching movement in this country. He knew all too well the horrors resulting from the denial of one's humanity and sense of dignity in Nazi Germany. He also noted the same type of oppression occurring in the African American inner-city school on Witherspoon Street in Princeton, New Jersey, in which he volunteered. Growing up in a poor community in Brooklyn, New York, I witnessed long lines of neighbors leading to fresh fruit and vegetable trucks that appeared weekly in my neighborhood. This was decades ago, and to see their reappearance as "new" health campaigns seems quite remarkable to me. In fact, I do not know why they went away in the first place!

Realize the Genius within Those You Serve

When we strip people of their social significance, we also bar the fruition of their hopes, dreams, and talents. Their potential accomplishments and contributions to their community, society, and possibly the world are forever lost. However, this goes further: they are stripped of their dignity. There comes a point when the wounds of morbidity and a premature mortality arise after outside parties cross the line of social dignity within these communities. Your attempts at intervention may, knowingly or unknowingly to you, cross this line as well. To be at all effective in such an environment, interventionists must understand this. Great harm can come to the recipient of a morally and ethically unsound intervention.

This requires one to break the institutionalized dogma so pervasive in general societal settings. One must actively unmask at a conscious level the invisible subpopulations. Engage and include all community members in planning efforts, and do not trivialize their input. Also realize that early intervention is critical to prevent long-term complications and consequences.

The gaps between the existing community infrastructure resources of a community and that which is required for an intervention plan to be successful must be ascertained. Failure to assess these discrepancies can result in the implementation of poorly planned and ineffective strategies. Both a worsening of the social situation and an accentuation of the feelings of helplessness can result from the implementation of a flawed and failed intervention strategy. This is especially true when it fails to address the underpinnings and root causes that gave rise to the disparities and injustices.

In the next chapter, I give a view of the insurance system that is based upon my personal experiences in dealing with insurance. This view represents my personal impressions of the medical insurance system. It raises the question of whether this is the best system under which the health care delivery system can operate.

Chapter 8

The Poorly Constructed Insurance System

I am not an expert in the insurance industry, and experts may disagree with my viewpoint on it. However, I have had many difficulties trying to understand the underpinnings of this industry on a logical, rational basis with what I currently know.

To my knowledge, the insurance system essentially began in Germany with injury claims from coal miners. If a coal miner was injured, he would sue his company in a tort claim action. The case would then take decades to resolve, leaving the person and his family to suffer. When the claim was settled, however, the company would have to pay out a large monetary settlement. As a result, the concept of strict liability arose. This was in the form of a compromise in which the company would assume liability for the worker's injury. The additional caveat was that the worker would be paid soon after the accident but at a capitated lesser amount of money. Thereby, both the injured worker who received his money earlier and the company that paid a lesser amount seemed to get a better deal.

Subsequently, in the United States, this concept was applied to homes and cars. There was an implied shared liability based on group membership with respect to risk-based outcomes. For example, suppose you have one million people paying one thousand dollars into a yearly homeowners' insurance system. If one home burns down, you have enough money to pay for the replacement of that one home. This is because the collective contributions made by the insurance policy owners created a shared liability risk pool of one billion dollars. In this circumstance, we can easily see how you can take care of or even replace a damaged home or car.

This shared liability model was applied to health care during a period of intense industrial development. It generally covered the development of serious medical illnesses that resulted in a long period of incapacitation or an untimely death. A shared risk pool covered those who were unfortunate enough to find themselves in these situations.

It is my view that a shared liability risk pool model does not adequately support the implementation of a medical treatment-based system in modern times in the United States. With the marked increase in unhealthy populations, the needs of the people covered are no longer met by a shared-risk system.

When hurricanes Katrina and Rita occurred, there were many insured homes damaged that were in the insurance risk pool. On average, people were not contributing payment amounts that would cover the rebuilding of all the homes that were affected. I envision that we are headed toward a similar outcome with respect to the health care insurance system as it is currently devised.

To decrease the relative risk of a poor outcome in such an insurance model, a prevention-centered approach is required. This must include an education-centered behavioral approach as well as a general screening and surveillance approach toward prevention and early detection of illness and disease. The elimination of unhealthy food products is also extremely important. Without an attempt to minimize poor outcomes through risk reduction or elimination, the insurance system will never be able to meet the needs of a flood of unhealthy individuals.

The Changing View about Health

There was also a dramatic shift with respect to the view of what being 'healthy' means. At the same time, there was a dramatic expansion of diagnostic and treatment modalities and options. For example, we found out that the standards we set and considered to be 'normal' were actually in some circumstances grossly abnormal. Cholesterol was falsely set at a very high 'normal value' level. It was initially based on a population of young and otherwise healthy and physically active military recruits. However, these recruits were consuming foods high in cholesterol when they were selected to set the cholesterol standards. This led to the false notion that their cholesterol levels were normal, and those levels were applied to the general population. Scientists shifted their perspective with respect to what it meant to be healthy.

After a surge in the recognition of cardiovascular disease was noted, scientists began not to accept the fact that people 'normally' die in their fifth and sixth decades of life. It was noted that people actually could live well into their eighth and ninth decades and beyond while maintaining a relatively pain-free and healthy state of being. The standards for cholesterol were then set at lower levels. Scientists recognized that behavior and dietary modifications resulted in a prolonged and improved quality of life.

With respect to the medical insurance system, the problem is that currently the share that each person pays into risk pool does not cover even basic tests. I speculate that if everyone who is insured were to come forward simultaneously to take all their required 'routine tests,' it would rapidly devastate and potentially bankrupt the insurance industry.

This industry is still basically operating on the antiquated risk-pool model. This is deeply problematic for an aging population riddled with multiple disease-related risk factors and a fundamentally transformed vision of what it means to be healthy. I feel that President Obama was exactly right, and visionary, when he proposed a universal health care system with a heavy focus on prevention.

The Need for a Wellness and Prevention Focus

It is imperative that a strong emphasis be placed upon the construction of wellness and preventative health systems. This must occur from both a cultural transformative and an individually-focused wellness and prevention standpoint.

COL. Damon T. Arnold, M.D., M.P.H.

It is essential to develop health-centered education curriculum in our academic institutions. This framework must establish the basis for a two-way communication mechanism that incorporates both individual and community member viewpoints into the intervention plan. For too long, the medical system has focused mainly on the provision of treatment services for preventable injuries, illnesses, and diseases—without setting the correct metrics or sufficiently engaging community members in health care prevention-focused discussions and education.

I often envision public health workers as people on a beach. They are standing on sand between those they would protect and at least two gigantic waves that threaten to crash upon them. One wave represents injuries, illnesses, and diseases, with obesity and substance abuse being prominent within this wave. The response to this should be focused on strongly supported and effective prevention interventions to combat this growing wave. The other wave represents a fragmented, underfunded, failing, and overburdened health care system. This latter wave is the treatment arm that is already under tremendous pressure to respond to and provide a safety net for the failing health of the general population.

Prevention also plays an extremely important role throughout the spectrum of treatment, regardless of the underlying stage of injury, illness, or disease that is present. Figure 3 illustrates this relationship. It identifies the decreasing effectiveness of prevention interventions, as one proceeds from Stage I to Stage IV disease, with a progressive increase in physical disability.

However, prevention can be leveraged across the injury, illness, and disease stages in an attempt to reduce the more costly consequences stemming from a purely treatment-focused approach. The inadequate treatment or unchecked advancement of these conditions imperils the entire health care system. Therefore, prevention also plays a direct role in the cost containment of the consequences of injuries, illnesses, and diseases by attempting to reduce poor medical management.

Resources must be allocated and directed at addressing the health status of the nation from a prevention-focused vantage point—that is, with respect to the avoidance of injuries, illnesses, and diseases as well as treatment should this become needed. To do less presages the appearance of the iceberg that sinks the health care ship.

As noted earlier, we cannot withstand the devastating impact of the wave of obesity and diabetes that is gaining strength throughout our nation and globally. Limited and localized treatment intervention strategies will provide little, if any, benefit in averting and mitigating the consequences arising from such a pervasive and massive population-based wave of ill health.

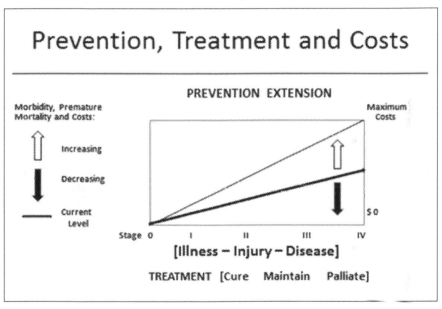

Figure 3. Stage I to Stage IV illness, injury, disease, and progressive physical disability over time. Further, the solid black diagonal line within the rectangle can move, as noted by the arrows, in an increasing or decreasing direction. If the prevention strategies are effective, the line will move in a decreasing direction, indicating a reduction in morbidity and premature deaths and overall health care costs. If it moves in an increasing direction, then morbidity and premature mortality increases, as do overall costs. The prevention arms represented by the vertical black arrow must be extended throughout the treatment spectrum.

Figure 3 does not illustrate the potential for what is denoted as the present cost level to dramatically increase with an overall less healthy and aging health care workforce. This makes the situation increasingly dire and heightens the call for immediate action. Further, we have a tendency to add up the true costs of an illness simply as being equivalent to the direct medical costs to the person afflicted. The cost of a heart attack is usually calculated simply as being equivalent to the ambulance ride, emergency department visit, angioplasty or bypass surgery, and the intensive, general, and rehabilitative care costs. It is then believed that this is the total cost. However, when looking further into this issue, one realizes that the ripple effect of this medical event involves not just a physical body stricken with heart disease. Rather, this person actually may have lost income, the possibility of future employment, or even the prospect of a pension.

If the person could not afford medical insurance, or even life insurance, she is now at risk of financial collapse. Her family may be on the brink of becoming homeless due to the loss of income. Her children may not be able to attend school, foreshadowing less potential for obtaining future education and gainful employment. This puts them all at risk for poor health and lost opportunities to achieve a higher degree of individual and family economic and social stability. They become entangled in the aftermath of poor health outcomes within the death spiral of disparity.

The Ripple Effects of Poor Health Impacts of an Individual upon the Community

In addition to the losses to the individual and her family members, community and workplace losses can occur. If she is unable to return to work or dies shortly after her heart attack, it may result in the loss of a supportive community member and a well-trained employee.

If the afflicted individual is a business owner or a person with a skill essential for the survival of the company, this may result in the loss of many jobs if the company were to go out of business. The social implications of the secondary and tertiary waves of disruption from a single individual stricken by the consequences of disease can be staggering. Contemplating the size of the obesity epidemic and the enormous resultant disease burden, one can clearly see that a high degree of social disruption would ensue.

So, an individual's injury, illness, or disease can cause dramatic tears in the social fabric of a family as well as society in general. This is especially true if that person has a pivotal, critical, or essential role in the creation of social and infrastructure stability for the community members involved. It is therefore essential that attempts to address health from a wellness and prevention intervention standpoint also involve a strong employer—and community-based social network.

In the next chapter, I present a social disruption model for interventionists to utilize in viewing various factors that contribute to individual and community stability and health.

Chapter 9

A Social Disruption Model for Interventionists

Social disruption can be approached with a conceptual model of my crafting that attempts to address public health concerns from a unified, comprehensive, and cohesive vantage point. This approach focuses upon essential and vitally important factors that support or disrupt the possibility of living a long and healthy life, individually or collectively.

A View of the Critical Infrastructure and Key Resource (CIKR) Sectors

The Department of Homeland Security has noted 17 CIRK sectors that support the population occupying a community area or region, as noted below in Figure 4.

Critical Infrastructure and Key Resource (CIKR) Sectors:	
1. Agriculture and Food	10. Energy
2. Banking and Finance	11. Government Facilities
3. Chemical	12. Information Technology
4. Commercial Facilities	13. National Monuments (Icons)
5. Commercial Nuclear	14. Postal and Shipping
6. Dams	15. Public Health and Health Care
7. Defense Industrial Base	16. Telecommunications
8. Drinking Water/Treatment	17. Transportation Systems
9. Emergency Services	

Figure 4. Critical Infrastructure and Key Resource (CIKR) sectors

In the spring of 2009, I sent a letter to the Department of Homeland Security (DHS) asking for *sanitation* to be included as a sector, as the collapse of this sector can have dire consequences from a public health perspective. This includes water treatment, raw sewage treatment, trash removal, and food safety and security systems. For example, a sanitation worker shortfall during a pandemic could open the door for the emergence of epidemics that could superimpose themselves upon the pandemic as well as the creation of animal and rodent control problems.

The sectors noted above are essential for ensuring community stability. They vary greatly in their functionality from region to region and range from supportive to disruptive and dysfunctional. As a result, they can provide support or impart harm to community members serviced by them. These sectors are directly related to the overall stability and functional status of the community they attempt to support.

There is also a general-population average level of stability (noted in Figure 5). For instance, at any given time, there are stabilizing factors such as a functional hospital or an after-hours ATM machine. However, there may also be a street light that is not functioning, someone driving without fastening his or her seat belt, and another person slipping on ice and falling. This average level of social order wavers and is affected by both man-made and environmental conditions and changes. However, a simple averaging across the entire general population tends to obscure the presence of underlying instabilities clustered within various subpopulations.

Subpopulations of Disparity and Relative Social Disruption Impacts

These subpopulations, noted in Figure 5, include people with increased morbidity and premature mortality associated statistically with membership within the various groupings or categories. For example, these categories can be denoted by race, ethnicity, gender, age, income, sexual orientation, a specific disability, religious affiliation, or geographic location.

Due to blatant ignorance, antisocial personality traits, and immorality, there are those that arise within society who attempt to attach illogical and erroneous stigmas to these various categories of social membership. They may even erroneously attach blame to these individuals for the various dire circumstances these victims find themselves within.

One can envision an impoverished community where a particular individual has a lack of access to education, employment, and health care while living in a food desert in an inner city or rural community. Such a subpopulation has a greater degree of vulnerability, instability, and resulting social disruption than the average person in the general population that surrounds them. An individual may also find himself or herself isolated or even explicitly prohibited from being present at or participating in activities in these general or private community domains.

This discrepancy can be viewed as the difference attributable to the term *disparity* and is denoted by the space between the special subpopulation and the general population lines depicted below in Figure 5. The graph plots the relative social disruption (RSD) level, or degree of social order present, against time.

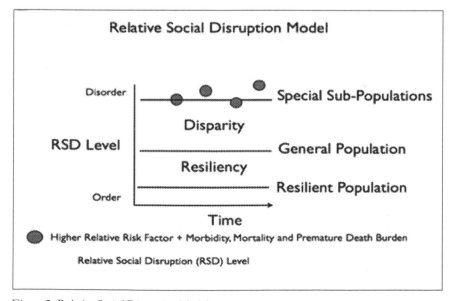

Figure 5. Relative Social Disruption Model

However, a food desert can exist even in a relatively affluent community in which social behaviors allow the consumption of high-calorie and less-than-nutritious meals. If a person routinely consumes five hot dogs and drinks six beers at a sporting event, he or she is at increased risk for the development of disease. That is, even if they live within an affluent community setting, their behavior is consistent with an unhealthy lifestyle, regardless of their socioeconomic status. When there are no healthy alternatives available in a setting, they are within a 'functional' food desert.

The term *disparity* implies a fundamental difference or inequality existing between two different groups of individuals. It is generally with respect to a resource or benefit because of their respective group memberships. This often arises from various forms of discrimination directed at a specific physical or social attribute that serves as the basis for a stigma-based lie. As mentioned earlier, there are many fallacies of logic, and they have a strongly dogmatic foothold in these types of situations. This dogma circulates within the gyroscope of geopolitics and socioeconomics. There is also an old saying that "absolute power concedes absolutely nothing."

Underlying factors resulting in this instability and giving rise to disparities are often systemic and can last for generations. To resolve such disparities, one must address the underlying dysfunctional social policies, beliefs, and practices in addition to CIKR sector inequalities. The increased social disruption occurring within these disparately impacted subpopulations can be eliminated only when a concerted effort is made to address the actual underlying root causes giving rise to the instability.

There are also disparity magnitude differences between the different subpopulation groups. This depends in great part on how many and to what degree various factors are present and what their combined effects are.

Holes in the Safety Net of Health

If social support systems are inadequate or dysfunctional, they tend to initiate and perpetuate morbidity and premature mortality. Underlying social disruption is distinct from the various physical conditions and agent exposures that become manifest. The conditions experienced by the impacted subpopulation are a reflection of poorly constructed and disruptive social policies. This also includes the social determinants of health as discussed earlier, based on various group memberships, such as race, gender, and age. For example, a person may eat foods high in trans-fats, cholesterol, and calories. This may be the result of a personal choice when alternatives exist or the result of the surrounding food desert, where no alternative choices exist. However, due to a person's race, gender, or age group, he or she may receive limited choices and suboptimal care should he or she be injured, become ill, or develop a disease. Such situations have been poorly documented in the literature and media. This is mainly because the people affected are generally poor and without effective political or collective social power.

It is possible to increase the relative general population's, or subpopulation's, stability and resiliency by increasing its resistance to change. This is denoted by the resilient population line in Figure 6. This objective can be accomplished through the strengthening of the underlying CIKR sectors and the elimination or mitigation of potential agent exposures and hazards within a community by imposing structural changes.

Attempts to engineer out such problems can be extremely effective but require adequate resource investments. This can also be accomplished through policy and practice changes within the various community sectors. At a minimum, this must also involve focused educational activities and the engagement of the community members themselves in the entire process.

Thus, community resilience shields the members from various degrees of morbidity and premature mortality. This is especially true should they face an unexpected change in conditions that puts them at increased risk for potential harm. An interventionist can provide education, training, and drills to the population potentially affected.

Conversely, it must be appreciated that the continued stability of inadequate systems that produce harm can be detrimental to the health outcomes of community members. Clearly, new approaches that herald the appearance of healthy outcomes need to be envisioned. They also need to be supported and implemented so that they replace antiquated models that continue to produce harm. These inadequate systems are more likely to fail during disasters as well, as we witnessed with Hurricane Katrina.

A concerted effort must also be focused upon both existing and potential problems to protect those at risk—with respect to agents arising within incidents or planned events that go awry which impose themselves upon the community infrastructure's functional baseline. Community buy-in and engagement facilitates not only the accomplishment of these goals but the development of community participant trust in the process as well.

Stability, Instability, and Relative Risk

A transition from one stability level to another, whether in a more stable or less stable direction, can be expressed in terms of a change in the relative risk for a particular outcome. The transition point is described as the meta-stable point where change can occur. In general, during a disaster, movement toward increased stability is associated with a decrease in the relative risk for a poor health outcome. A movement toward decreased stability (instability) is generally associated with an increase in the risk of a poor health outcome.

Note also that there is a logarithmic increase in social disruption as an individual or population transitions from one level to a higher level of instability. This increase can be as a result of various additive and synergistic effects. These effects arise from the combination and interaction among various social determinants and the CIKR sector factors and causative agents that may act to potentiate each other. It may also occur because of a lack of sufficient resources to compensate for the encountered disruptive forces.

An individual may have several risk factors, such as heart disease, poor nutritional habits, and cigarette smoking. It is not just simply a matter of adding these risk factors together to arrive at a neat mathematical sum of combined impacts. Rather, each of these factors complicates the other factors involved and results in a much more dire and complicated situation. This is especially true when they potentiate each other. An individual may not just face a mathematical sum of his or her risk factors leading to poor health. In reality he or she may be contending with geometrically worsening health because of the combination of the specific factors present. Also, infrastructure failures may combine to produce a worsening situation on a geometric scale. This will make the situation at hand much more difficult to contend with.

Considerations in Establishing Priorities for Intervention

A reflection upon the various risk factors can determine which of these factors should be addressed first and in what order. To eliminate their destructive combinatorial effects most effectively, one must understand how the various factors are related and operate within the context of an individual's life or the general population.

This must be done with the intention of minimizing and mitigating the expected and emerging morbidity and premature mortality. Consideration must be given to the relative contribution that each risk factor's presence portends—for the future health of the exposed individual as well as the population at large. Attention must also be given to ensuring that harm is not imparted to the person being helped by the intervention process itself. Care must be taken in the selection, ordering, and timing of the risk factors that need to be addressed.

Instability Treads upon a Geometric Path

Individuals have varying degrees of an innate resiliency that is closely aligned with their basic survival skills. However, the space that exists between the general population and the resilient population lines on the graph is reflective of 'acquired' resiliency. This requires the development of skills or responses to anything from the minor problems one encounters to life-threatening, full-scale disasters.

As depicted in Figure 6, "Stability-Instability Vacillations and the Social Disruption Model," these incidents and destabilized events fall along a logarithmic scale. This scale ranges from minor increases in instability to the occurrences of disastrous proportions and consequences. In explaining the components of Figure 6, I will start from the bottom and then work toward the top.

Individual and collective community social behaviors are noted at the bottom of the graph. This level represents a listing of some of the most salient factor categories for the social structure and networking within a community. These factors include things such as prevailing myths, beliefs, philosophies, and dogmas. These arise from perceptions and views concerning morals, ethics, personal integrity, and values held by the community members themselves.

These various views can be associated with both positive and negative outcomes for each individual or the community as a whole. For example, these factors can be directed at the provision of stabilizing influences with resources directed at mutually beneficial projects. With good intentions and a spirit of collaboration, one can gain an accurate, logical assessment of social needs. This can result in the establishment of community trust and heightened stability directed toward the betterment of community members.

The aforementioned views can also result in general, subpopulation, and even individual negative impacts. This can result from the imposition of policies based on bad intent, misrepresentations, fallacies, or self-interest that lead to negative social consequences for the involved community members. The disruptive forces that arise within a community originate, only in part, in the morals, ethics, values, and integrity-based viewpoints of community members. Disruptive forces within a community can also have a basis in the geopolitical and socioeconomic underpinnings imposed upon a community by an external group. Negative impacts can also result from the application of inappropriate interventions based on poor planning, miscalculations, and thoughts based upon fallacious logic.

Figure 6 illustrates the relationship between various levels of social stability as they occur within a community. The occurrence of a natural or man-made disaster further destabilizes the general population (GP) and the impacted subpopulations (SP), although to vastly different degrees.

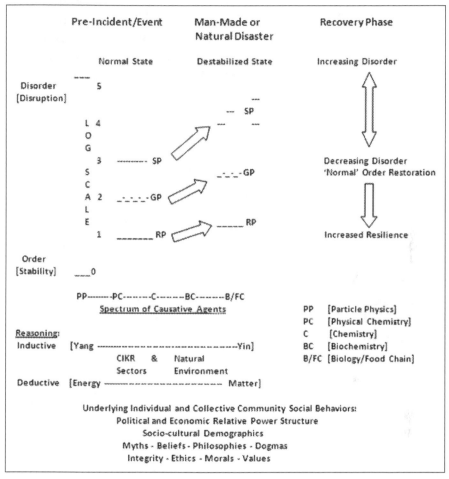

Figure 6. Stability-Instability Vacillations and the Social Disruption Model

The relative power contained within a community's political and economic infrastructures is extremely important for the maintenance and restoration of social order. The model illustrates that communities require more resources for recovery from not only everyday living but also from disasters and deleterious event. The degree of displacement is experienced on a logarithmic scale. The further displaced the community population or subpopulation becomes, the more difficult it is to meet the attendant needs of community members on a geometric scale.

Should disasters repeatedly occur in an area, it is wise for community planners to develop transitional community recovery models. These models should support the establishment of more stable and health-focused community infrastructures as attempts are made to rebuild. This should involve a high degree of community member involvement and could solve some of the problems that existed in the community infrastructure even before the occurrence of a subsequent disaster.

As a result, the combined effects of risk factors lead to a geometric worsening of the infrastructure situation. This implies that more effort and resources need to be applied to resolve what may appear at first glance to be an isolated issue. One may get the impression that the task at hand is resource intensive, even for getting simple tasks accomplished. This may be because of a lack of focus on the larger picture as well as the interrelationship between the factors complicating the response efforts.

The relative level of disruption experienced within a community should be approached from a process mapping perspective. The relative urgency of various problems should be determined. The problems should be looked at in a holistic fashion. This requires a paradigm shift from a more traditionally Western way to an Eastern way of viewing the environment. This aligns nicely with various aspects of the green environments and technologies movements occurring within this country. This should also be kept in mind when contemplating rebuilding efforts.

Critical Infrastructure and Key Resource (CIKR) Sectors and the Internal Environment

The next level in Figure 6 describes the CIKR sectors and the natural environment level. This includes the man-made resources that comprise the CIKR sectors listed. Further, these are superimposed upon the natural environment. The community environment is the setting in which the social order arises. It reflects the societal forces that both forged and continue to maintain its existence. This serves as the environment, a mixture of natural and man-made conditions, in which communities exist. This environment dramatically varies on a geographic basis and over time as one transitions from community to community.

This level of the diagram contains the entire energy-matter spectrum of agents contained within a community. All of the agents that can be used for the betterment or worsening of social order arise from this spectrum. The spectrum contains everything from particle physics to the food chain. Particle physics includes both the safe production of nuclear energy to the devastatingly negative impacts of nuclear weapons. Likewise, the food chain includes the production of healthy organic foods as well as the creation of trans fats, which cause heart disease. Agents along this spectrum can be used with good or bad outcomes, as they can lead to social cohesion and stability or the advent of poor health and instability, respectively. What is important is how and in which ways we choose to deal with the use of these man-made and natural environmental agents and resources.

The Disparate Impact of Disruption

The next level in Figure 6 relates to the relative degree of social order or disorder. Depicted here are the resilient, general, and disparately impacted subpopulations within a community.

These groupings are initially shown during periods when there is a 'normal' background level of social order. This is then followed by a period of a relatively heightened level of disruption. The period of heightened disruption occurs after an incident or miss-event has caused a higher degree of social disorder. Subsequent to this, a period of recovery is noted.

I chose to represent the relative scale of social order and disorder as logarithmic. Again, the social determinants of health and societal factors cannot simply be added together in a linear, mathematical fashion to determine the degree of benefit or harm imparted by an incident or miss-event. One will be misled by the use of a linear, tabular scale or checklist to discern the impacts of various risk factors in a community. One must determine the relevance and combined effects of various risk factors to arrive at an assessment of the impact(s).

Risk factors interact to form geometric, antagonistic, additive, and synergistic effects on an individual or community as a whole. I use the logarithmic scale to demonstrate that recovery from a higher state of imposed disorder may require a geometrically larger amount of resources and skills to assist an individual or community in need of help in returning to its baseline state of social order.

Figure 6 depicts the impact of an incident or miss-event that works to further destabilize a resilient, general, or disparately impacted subpopulation. Figure 7 further describes the community impacted by an incident or event.

Recovery from any disaster must also be viewed from the vantage point of the level of innate preparedness and resiliency within a community. The underlying, relative community stability, based upon its innate levels of preparedness and resiliency, is an important indicator of a community's recovery potential.

Resiliency has at least two basic components. The first is resistance to change in the face of internal or external influences. The second is the ability to rebound from a point of relative displacement once the negatively impacting factors have diminished, completely subsided, or been actively extinguished.

The more affluent sectors of the general population have more rebound resiliency than disparately impacted subpopulations. They have access to more resources and political will to forge a road to the recovery and restabilization of their communities.

Disparately impacted communities become the fodder of unscrupulous media-driven frenzies—a "what bleeds, leads" mentality. But when the images of community members slip into obscurity, the sound-bite loses its corporate media worth. However, most media sources have greatly improved in this regard and have become allies in this battle. One of the best at this new supportive approach is CNN. Several local channels have recently followed suit. Public television has always been visionary and balanced in this regard.

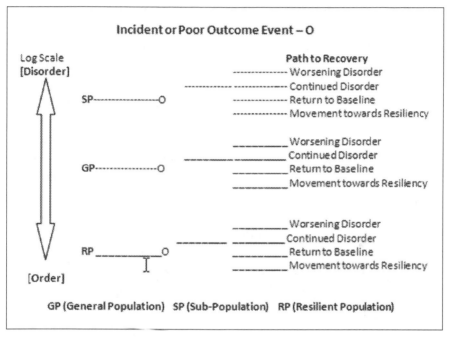

Figure 7. Incident or poor outcome events and the path to recovery

Disparately impacted subpopulations may initially display remarkable intrinsic resiliency, abilities in adaptation, and coping skills. These arise from routine attempts to overcome the social realities and inequities they face daily within their already disrupted and unstable community settings.

These inequities become evident as the lack of proper and sufficient infrastructure support mechanisms unfolds and systemic failures ensue. However, once these disparately impacted community members face limited and dwindling resources, the edge of their cliff of their response capabilities is reached. All too often society has stood witness to the fact that resiliency, adaptability, and coping can topple. The sustainability of efforts, directed at community re-stabilization, depends mostly upon access to the resources required to meet the needs of community members. If one assumes these individuals can deal with hard times and "take care of themselves," tragic results will materialize as they decompensate.

The line SP represents sub-populations that have been impacted by shared social determinants or demographic features. A member of the impacted community need not share all of the characteristics associated with other members of the community to be affected. The aggregate effect of the features present results in a disparate impact within the community. This affects all of those who are community members and even visitors.

The more resilient populations (RP) can still experience an increase in relative instability. However, they are more resistant to becoming disordered or displaced. This group generally has access to resources that the disparately impacted communities do not. Also, the digital divide still exists within disparately impacted communities. Hopefully, as technology advances, it offers hope for the educational and communication access requisite for the development of community-based resiliency.

A disaster superimposed itself upon the normal background level and intensifies the relative disorder within the affected community. However, it will have a varied effect on the various societal component levels represented by the resilient, general, and disparately impacted subpopulations. The disparately impacted subpopulations will be affected to a greater degree, on a geometrically increasing scale, than the general population—with respect to a disproportionately higher degree of resultant pain, suffering, and premature deaths.

Comments on the Path to Recovery

To restabilize a community, risk factors must be considered both individually and collectively. One must understand how agent risk factors operate to determine their contribution to the outcome. It is important in determining which, and in what order, the factors should be addressed. If the factors contributing the most to the heightened level of instability can be correctly identified, their removal should cause a faster rate, and possibly greater degree, of recovery. This is especially true for the more geometrically destabilized and disparately impacted communities.

A formal review of risk factor interactions is beyond the scope of this book. However, one can glean a basic understanding of how factors may interact to produce various outcomes through a review of some basic principles of chemistry. I have listed the definitions of various effects arising from chemical mixture interactions below.

Additive: The additive effects of two or more chemicals when combined is equal to each of their individual effects added together. This is analogous to adding 2 + 2 to get 4.

Synergistic: The effects of two or more chemicals when combined is greater than the simple arithmetic sum of their individual effects. This is analogous to adding 2 + 2 and getting 10 as the result.

Antagonistic: The effects of two or more chemicals when combined is less than the sum of their individual effects. This is analogous to adding 2 + 2 and getting 3 as a result.

Potentiation: This is when a chemical with no effect itself enhances or promotes the effect of another chemical agent. This is analogous to adding 0 + 2 to get 7.

Coalitive: This is when factors that have no effects of their own when added together result in an effect. This is analogous to adding 0 + 0 to get 5.

From a simple review of these principles, one can begin to glean an understanding of how various risk factors may interact to produce sometimes unexpected outcomes. For instance, a dilapidated building may contain asbestos in its basement walls. If occupants of the building try to clean this up without training or guidance, they are at increased risk of a significant exposure to asbestos. This increases their risk of mesothelioma, a cancer of the membranes that cover the lungs. If, however, they are also cigarette smokers, they geometrically increase their risk for cancer. This is because asbestos and cigarette smoke are synergistic with respect to the risk for developing this form of cancer. Their individual effects are not simply additive, but result in a greatly increased risk for cancer. This is essentially also true for the various risk-factor agents encountered in community-based settings—that is, whether they are of an energy-matter, geopolitical, or social policy origin.

After a community experiences a natural or man-made disaster, several outcomes are possible. Figure 7 illustrates that a community can initially stabilize at a higher level of disorder only to face the worsening of this condition. This can become manifest with a passage of time in which there is the depletion of the resources required to accomplish full recovery. For example, after the earthquakes in Haiti, community members in the affected regions faced the consequences of having a higher degree of imposed disorder. This included having no shelter, poor sanitation, and a lack of access to food. This would then precipitate conditions ripe for potential infectious disease outbreaks and societal collapse. This was also very apparent with Hurricanes Katrina and Rita in New Orleans, Louisiana. One cannot simply look at the factors involved without realizing that they are extremely interactive and interdependent. This underscores the need for a rational comprehension of how these factors work together to move either towards further instability or the recovery of community-based stability.

Additional Comments on Social Disruption

In summary, one cannot view all communities in the same light. There should be a concerted effort to increase the resiliency and preparedness levels of all communities in the United States. This is essential to ensure community survival when confronted by a catastrophic incident or event that goes awry.

Further, the social conditions that underlie disparately impacted communities make them much more vulnerable to the threats of both man-made and natural disasters—on a geometric rather than an arithmetic progression scale. This higher level of instability can require more resources and services in order to restore community stability. The relative degree of disorder is eerily analogous to quantum mechanics applied to the electron shell theory in chemistry—that is, when describing the geometrically based magnitudes of relative energy as one passes from one quantum shell level to another.

At this juncture I must underscore the need to strengthen infrastructures within these communities from both a preparedness and resiliency standpoint. This requires political will and fiscal investments in these communities that all too often are lacking, if not absent all together.

In the next chapter, I present some views interventionists may want to contemplate as they approach social disruptions within a community environment. This is only a starting point for the internal dialogue interventionists must face within themselves as they interact with the community members for which they provide service.

Chapter 10

The Interventionist's Approach to Social Disruption

Response roles for interventionists during social disruptions can be quite varied, whether arising from usual social instability, man-made or natural disasters, or miss-events. However, there are some basic principles that apply to all responders upon entering a socially disrupted setting.

The Role of the Public Health Interventionist

Often people recently entering the field of medicine, public health, or military medical services ask me what their first step should be. I draw a curve on a piece of paper that covers all the people in the region they intend to work with—whether on a national, state, or local level. I then tell them to handpick a single point from beneath the curve.

They are then told that the point they picked represents a person. At this point they are instructed to "erase" the person's gender, age, race, ethnicity, social status, sexual orientation, educational level, and geographic origin. Any other identifiable features that distinguish this person from the other points under the curve are also removed. Once this is accomplished, they must then realize that what they are holding in their hand is the essence of a miraculous human life. It is no different from any other point under the curve.

Next they are to realize the factors that are causing pain, suffering, and premature death for the individual being serviced. The interventionist must provide aid in the resolution of these issues and attempt to prevent negative health consequences from impacting this individual. He or she must do his or her best, using the resources at hand, to address disparities observed between any of these points. This is a position of equality for those being serviced. Such a view may be supported by moral and ethical codes, religious doctrine, or legal parlance. The interventionist must, however, recognize it as the inalienable, essential, and miraculous condition of being a human being on this earth.

The Application of Resources

You should professionally apply your skills, abilities, and resources based solely upon the relative needs of the population members. The allocation of resources should mirror where the individual burdens of pain, suffering, and the potential for an earlier-than-expected demise exist. This is when you have the correct perspective for implementing population-based strategies—that is, for improving health and preventing pain, suffering, and premature deaths within the entire population you are covering.

In addition, if any individual is ignored due to any of the factors in the example above, you further increase their pain, suffering, and risk for premature death. This also weakens the community's social infrastructure. That is legally, constitutionally, ethically, and morally inconsistent with the foundational principles of public health practice. Such an approach also provides fertile soil for the perpetuation of social disparities. In essence, such an orientation works in support of the perpetuation of social disorder, injustice, and the resultant pain, suffering, and premature death. Do not tread upon this path or assist anyone so inclined. We must not work in a direction that alienates other human beings.

It should be noted that this abhorrent behavior works on behalf of the creation of potential nodal points for the emergence of antisocial and even terroristic behavioral patterns. The emergence of such behaviors might arise as a reaction to being disenfranchised on the part of those recipients of discriminatory acts. This reaction threatens not only community stability, but national and global security as well.

One must adhere to the basic tenants of a professional, competent, ethical, morally sound, just, and respectful approach to any individual who is in need. If one cannot comply with this essential requirement, one's first step should be outside the practice of medicine and public health. The person who can comply with these basic tenants should be welcomed to the profession with open arms. Those who hold these ideals and utilize the best public health practices on both scientific and humanistic levels should provide guidance to these new public health workers.

In *Chapter 3—The Relationship Which Dwells Within,* I explained my CLAM'N model. An interventionist must guard against the development of conflict which results in coercion or the need for litigation, arbitration, and mediation. One must learn to negotiate with community partners successfully while setting realistic expectations related to desired outcomes for all parties involved. There also must be respect for established boundaries and deep respect for another person's wishes.

An assessment must be made with respect to your perceptions of the balance of the order and disorder that underpin the environment you have entered. You must become attuned to and have a situational awareness of the social order and constructs as well as the inherent rhythms by which the community operates. Learn who is in power and who has influence over this community. To have an impact, you must have both acceptance and support from the community you are providing a service within. You will learn a great deal more than you teach. You will also gain a great deal more than you give, if your approach and service provision is correctly applied.

In the next chapter, I describe the concept of relative risk by using the coin-toss model. This approach to probability is an attempt to explain the relationship between relative order and disorder within a community setting.

Chapter 11

The Coin Toss of Order and Disorder

U ltimately, it is important to note that what is currently occurring within a community is not just a reflection of what is going on in the present. Rather, these communities have a history and collective cultural orientation toward a future state of being, as reflected in their community visions, policies, and practices. We all must take care with how this future will be carved out and under whose direction this process will occur. Both random and deliberative social forces can alter and become determinative with respect to the destiny of community members, despite their wishes.

The Weighting of the Probability Coin

Imagine a coin on which one side represents social order and the other social disorder. If you were to flip it, you have an equal chance of getting either order or disorder. However, what if the coin could be weighted in the direction of either order or disorder? You would change the odds of the relative risk. You would also, on the average, win most coin tosses.

In the context of a community setting, if the social circumstances are weighted toward the development of poor social outcomes and poverty, you will see the terrifying manifestations that arise from this orientation. For example, you may see excess morbidity and premature mortality, food deserts, dilapidated buildings, staggering unemployment, gang activity, violence, and rampant drug abuse. Also, note that if the community structure is slanted toward social disorder, the entire community becomes involved in the outcome. As with the example of a weighted coin, it is not possible to have half of a coin involved in the outcome. The entire coin is involved. The entire society will move as a whole, even if there are segregated compartments in operation within the community at large. If the community moves in the direction of disorder, the entire society will suffer the consequences of the decisions made in the weighting of the 'community coin.'

This weighting of the community coin can be viewed as the introduction of positive, cohesive movements toward order or of negative, disruptive movements toward social disorder. The weighting can also be affected by introduced changes in a community over time, whether of natural or man-made origin.

The Application of the Coin Toss Concept to the Environment

From either Eastern or Western philosophical viewpoints, this energy (yang) and matter (yin) balance can be viewed as a continuum which is affected by change. It is not that energy or matter is good or bad. Rather, it is whether the influences they produce result in positive or negative outcomes.

What ultimately matters is how these energy-matter relationships are envisioned, implemented, and transformed to create the surrounding physical and social environment. For example, it is important to ascertain what products are being created by and emanate from manipulations of the environment and utilized community resources. Determining how the availability of these products affects the community members themselves is extremely important. If they impart a greater degree of social disruption, they tend to raise the level of overall individual and community dysfunction, morbidity, and tendency toward premature mortality.

How they are envisioned and transformed is directed by the collective actions and conscious inputs of society as a whole. This involves not merely the energy we put into arranging our material world. It also involves how we have consciously chosen to accomplish this task and the results that are borne from our decisions. We are ultimately responsible for the environment we live in through our collective actions directed at the creation of social and environmental order or disorder. This begins with how we have conceptualized and directed the construction of the world we live in. It also involves our collective material impacts as well as the indirect systemic effects we produce.

Care must be taken in not to ascribe the social conditions witnessed in impoverished communities to community members that live there. The very presence of such manifestations often is the result of societal factors that resulted in a disparate impact on these community members. This is often based upon the unjust, immoral, and unethical behaviors of groups who exploit these communities from an external vantage point. In essence, such external groups weight the coin toward the production of social disorder and then blame the community members affected by the disparate conditions which arise from the fateful weighting of the coin. This also occurs while the group imparting this disorder in the affected community benefits in some way, often monetarily, from its imposition.

Progressive companies have been able to impart more order as a result of their business-related activities. Such actions leave communities in a better situation than when the progressive company first entered. For example, companies that provide fresh fruits and vegetables or safe exercise facilities and open spaces can provide the access required to ensure healthy community-oriented lifestyles.

In the next chapter, the battleground between community realities and scientific approaches to problem resolution is explored. I will use the concept of a bridge to explain the divide between the design of interventions produced purely on a scientific basis and the ultimate acceptance of a community intervention.

Chapter 12

Crossing the Battleground of the How?—Why? Bridge

P articipating as a colonel in the Army National Guard, I had the opportunity and honor of assisting in the efforts in Louisiana during hurricanes Katrina and Rita. Upon arrival, we moved into the field to treat survivors of this horrific disaster.

While walking in the ninth ward, I was struck by a realization, as if it were a lightning bolt. It occurred to me that people were asking questions from very different perspectives. I call it the battleground of the How?–Why? bridge.

The Footprints of the Bridge

To engage with a community, one must acknowledge the existence of the How?–Why? bridge. *How?* is a question for which science must provide an answer. Science notes the principles and mechanisms by which diseases are spread or treated, cars run, planes fly, or buildings should be built. The scientific method determines whether a hypothesis is valid or invalid. It is an approach based on logic and the use of an inductive or deductive reasoning process.

The people I met that survived the disaster never asked me the question "How did this happen?" Rather, they asked, "*Why* is this happening to us?" I immediately realized that this question stems from a religious, philosophical, socioeconomic, or geopolitical vantage point. That is, there was a major hurdle for the implementation of any form of intervention plan based purely on a mechanistic, scientific approach.

One must consider ideological explanations, opinions, and debatable viewpoints. One must understand the community culture and perspectives in order to be effective in community interventions. This is true whether they are delivered on a routine or emergent basis. Many times I have witnessed community intervention programs that totally disregard this fundamental issue. Also, the rights of individuals must be safeguarded. I have included a copy of the first ten amendments to the Constitution, the Bill of Rights, in appendix C of this book. Read them and protect against their potential erosion. Also, it is not a question of taking care of their problems over there but rather taking care of our problems over here.

There is a direct incongruence between the questions How? and Why? with respect to how they are being answered. This can result in miscommunication and an immediate and direct rejection by the proposed recipient of the service of the intervention to be employed. Interestingly, these interventions are called "community engagement programs." For an *engagement* to be valid, there has to be the acceptance and consent of the other party.

The People on the Other Side of the Bridge

The familiarity, comfort, and stability sought by those who find themselves in these situations are not just based on overcoming the physical environment. It is intertwined with their heredity, past experiences, surrounding cultural paradigms, and the social order of the environment they wish to restore.

Cultural myths and mores may be present and confronted within a community. However, they may serve as a source of protection against the recurrence of past transgressions. These intrusions may be viewed as personal assaults by the community members in question. The point is that these beliefs may protect of the community members involved and should not be lightly dismissed.

We are all physical, emotional, mental, and spiritual beings. In addition, in each of us is a balance between independence and a need to be alone, and a need for social interaction and togetherness. The attention we pay to each of our needs on this level can wax and wane. We must respect these boundaries with others during ordinary times and at times of crisis. Ignoring them will lead any intervention attempts down a path to noncompliance and potentially tragic outcomes.

This is why I have always asked anyone requesting a grant if they can answer the question 'Why?,' not as posed by me or them, but as presented by the intended recipients of the proposed intervention. "Why should I listen to you and change my behavior and place my trust in you and your intervention?"

You can have a scientifically sound method for mitigating pain, suffering, and premature death. However, if you have a crucible with a scientifically designed elixir that could cure all of humankind's ills, it means nothing if no one is willing to drink it. You might as well spill it onto the ground. If no one is willing to take it, what good does it do? To make it an effective intervention, you must know, respect, and understand the viewpoints of the recipients on the other side of the bridge—that is, the community members for which you are providing a service.

You Really Need to Understand the Dilemma

Always remember that the How?—Why? question arises within the context in which this person lives. This may involve the presence of a high degree of endemic social disruption or an improving or worsening state of social order. These circumstances may geometrically compound the problems they experience. For example, a parent may have a sick child. He may have an old car that has broken down. The medical facility he usually goes to is shut down. While seeking alternative transportation, he realizes that he is forced to take his child to another local establishment for care. But at this treatment facility he was once told, "*We do not take care for your uninsured kind.*" And he is unable to read, having access only to poor educational opportunities. There is no food, water, or medication available. It is easy to see how overwhelming circumstances can get in short order.

The understanding of these circumstances and the ability to respond with appropriate and effective interventions are essential for a positive outcome. This process is especially facilitated if social circumstances are clearly understood prior to the occurrence of a disaster, emergency, or event that goes awry. A lack of such an understanding will greatly complicate and hinder the success of any intervention strategy, whether of emergent or non-emergent origin.

Answer the Questions and Meet the Needs

The required elements of any intervention plan include ingredients such as competency, reliability, consistency, and above all, compassion on the part of the interventionist. The intervention must meet the physical, emotional, and psychological needs of all affected community members in a timely and sensitive manner. The spiritual nature of those afflicted with disparate impacts must be recognized as well. This may be a crucial aspect of life for some community members.

Be aware that discriminatory actions and behaviors, unconscious biases, and stereotyping by interventionists can influence the actual perception and analysis of the situation. This will have an impact on the intervention strategy employed, compliance by participating community members, and the intervention outcome. This form of interaction not only affects the individual involved in a negative fashion. It also can perpetuate feelings of fear and mistrust throughout the disparately impacted subpopulation. It is not the interventionist that determines all the parameters and metrics of a successful outcome, but the community members themselves. It is important to address the existing needs, but we must also have an accurate impression of what the community members want and how they define success.

Communicating with Blinders On

During the H1N1 pandemic response in the spring 2009, I paid close attention to what was being noted about the community responses to the vaccination campaign that was launched. I remember talking with my colleagues on the national, state, and local levels about the refusal of community members to accept the vaccine.

This was illogical when seen in relation to the prevailing scientific sense of logic at the time. After all, the vaccine was scientifically sound, protected against the onset of a potentially fatal illness, and was free. The answer to the scientific question 'How?' was apparent. The prevailing consensus of interventionists was that if a person turned down the vaccine, it must be because of a mythical belief or illogically derived conclusion on his or her part.

Some people turning down the vaccine thought that they could get the flu from eating pork or taking the vaccine. Others believed that thiomersol, present in doses of the vaccine, causes autism. Yet others thought it was some form of experimentation. These beliefs were held by both affluent and impoverished community members. It is important to note that such views do not correlate with the lack of education on the parts of those who hold them to be true.

Although some of these beliefs were present, they did not explain community-based viewpoints in a very large number of situations I had encountered. I began to think of the industrial workers that I have provided care to over many decades. This then led me to think of another plausible explanation.

One may approach a laborer who has a spouse and two young children about the need for vaccination. Suppose that the laborer works fourteen hours a day and sometimes even weekends. Further, this laborer went to the emergency room a month ago, as he was not feeling well, and he was found to have hypertension and diabetes. His wife, who accompanied him, seeing the opportunity, decided to get checked as well. She was found to have a breast mass. At the end of the encounter, he was told to follow up with his provider, at which point he mentioned the lack of insurance for himself or his wife. They then told him to go to a local health department, which was thirty miles away and open from 9:00 a.m. to 4:00 p.m. He said he could not comply with that and was given no other options, as he was uninsured.

This having occurred before he was asked about the flu shots for him and his family. He then inquired if there were any side effects and was told that there was a very small chance of an allergic reaction or a need for hospitalization. He flatly refused the vaccination. Not knowing what had transpired earlier in the emergency room, the provider was convinced that he either did not understand the science or was operating according to a mythical construct.

Actually, from the laborer's viewpoint, this was a rational choice. That is, he realized that he had no insurance or access to hospital care, which would come at a great cost. If he were to get sick from the vaccine, he would likely become hospitalized and unemployed, hurting his family directly. Further, he had not been treated for his diabetes or hypertension. Since the time of their emergency department visit, he and his wife had been examining her breast mass, fearfully checking for an increase in size.

Clearly we need to do much more work in this arena before assuming people just do not understand or are operating with a mythical belief system. There must be a concerted effort to recognize and address the individual and community perspectives as one attempts to cross the How?—Why? bridge. To ignore this element, or to transform it into an erroneous impression by incorrectly interpreting it, can result in intervention failure and individual and community member harm. A key component of intervention success is learning what is important to an individual or community—from their perspective, not yours.

The Health Treatment System Faces Prevention

Unfortunately, the health care system in this country has been heavily invested in battling the occurrence of injury, illness, and disease states, almost exclusively from a treatment perspective. In my experience, the concepts that guided the medical community toward the creation of prevention modalities were dogmatically blocked and vilified by those who professed to be medical experts.

You were not even allowed to bring the topic of prevention up—unless you wanted to face the wrath and scorn of dogmatic torchbearers who would proclaim you were attempting to practice witchcraft. I witnessed many a visionary senior residents or attending physician face the impalement tools of their closed-minded colleagues. It is amazing to witness some of these closed-minded colleagues now extolling the current prevention principles they decried in the past – and as if they were their very own from the beginning. This is disingenuous, at best.

Actually, the concepts of prevention and wellness have their origins in health practices that span thousands of years. The cradle of science in the Middle East and Africa gave rise to many of the holistic modalities practiced today. Several of the societies have vanished as the result of war or an externally imposed genocide perpetrated by invading colonial societies.

Well, thankfully, the holistic movement tied to principles of nutrition and Eastern concepts of prevention and treatment has thrived despite this immoral assault. Fortunately, I was able to learn concepts related to Eastern philosophy during my martial arts, massage therapy, and acupuncture training over many decades. I have found many of these modalities to be effective and supportive of general health—for both treatment and prevention when applied by well-trained practitioners.

One should be cautious and find professionals well trained in these arts, as there are many who claim to know them—likely after briefly reading a document that is the intellectual equivalent of a comic book. "*Caveat emptor!*" ("Buyer, beware!") Any such approach should also include the advice of an appropriately and competently trained Western practitioner. I see the Eastern and Western practitioners as allies in the practice of health care. Like anything else, each philosophy has its positives and negatives.

As noted earlier, proper and healthy nutrition is fundamental to having a healthy life. I have included several references in the bibliography as recommendations for you to use to explore and learn about the vast array of concepts and modalities for prevention in Eastern medicine. Despite your viewpoint on Eastern medicine, it is important to understand, as it is now a part of our culture. It is increasingly becoming entrenched within the communities you will enter.

COL. Damon T. Arnold, M.D., M.P.H.

Prevention must not be viewed just as a way to prevent the occurrence of injury, illness, and disease. Rather, it must also be extended throughout the treatment of injury, illness, and disease irrespective of stage.

The major point here is that we can no longer afford to orient the application of medical system resources and services from a viewpoint purely directed at treatment. The use of preventive health measures must be used throughout the continuum of routine life and with any degree of required medical care.

In *Part 4*, I transition to the topic of resiliency. This encompasses the innate resistance to change within a community when faced with disruptive forces. I will also discuss the ability to mitigate the possibility of ongoing harm within a disrupted environmental setting.

PART 4

The Development of Resiliency

Why Jack Died and Jill Did Not

The real reason for Jack's
terrible demise
was not his clumsiness
or foreboding size.
Rather, when he fell down
breaking his crown
it was simply because
he neglected to put on
the helmet of prevention.
Jill, being more wise,
having been trained to be more agile,
respected the safety helmet's invention.
She wore the helmet without safety rival
and experienced a milder fall
resulting in her ultimate survival.

— Damon T. Arnold, MD

Chapter 13

NIMS and the Need for Preparedness

Truely, never before has it been more important to have an interdisciplinary approach to preparedness. In part, this is due to the availability of historical and newer agents that are potentially harmful. One must also consider global terrorist threats and the occurrence of both man-made and natural disasters. In addition, due to the development of effective countermeasures, early warning systems, and rescue mechanisms, the chances for an individual's survival have dramatically increased.

What follows is a very brief overview of some key points concerning the National Incident Management System (NIMS). It must be stressed that this is just an overview of some of the more salient points regarding NIMS. It is not intended to replace a formal course of instruction on NIMS. Further, I strongly advise the reader to take the formal online training available at the www.fema.gov website. In addition, you must stay current. There are many excellent references available on this subject, some of which appear in the resources section of this book.

A Brief Overview of the ICS and NIMS

With the unfolding of recent disaster incidents and disrupted events, it is apparent that being prepared is not only recommended but essential. Being prepared in fact can be the determining factor between surviving intact and the onset of chronic pain and suffering or a premature death. Further, this preparedness orientation must be present on the individual, family, and community levels.

The National Incident Management System (NIMS) was created in response to the 9/11 terrorist attacks. It embodies decades of Incident Command System (ICS) based emergency response 'lessons learned' and the successful integration of established best business practices. It sets the basis for a coordinated approach to resource management and mutual aid among multiple disciplines and jurisdictions.

Prior to NIMS, the ICS was based on Department of Defense (DoD) principles. It was created in reaction to wildfire response failures in California in the 1970s, when unnecessary deaths and property damage occurred. The ICS was created in response to the identified lack of the proper management and coordination of that emergency response. In cooperation with ICS, NIMS allows for the bridging of complex single or multijurisdictional incidents or events that go awry. This provides a standardized, coordinated management approach and is based on the use of best practices for emergency, disaster, and disrupted event response efforts.

The Incident Command System is directed at facilitating response activities through five major functional areas: command, operations, planning, logistics, and finance/administration. Listed below are the 14 essential ICS features:

1. Modular Organization
2. Reliance on an Incident Action Plan (IAP)
3. Management by Objectives
4. Chain of Command and Unity of Command
5. Common Terminology
6. Deployment
7. Unified Command
8. Predesignated Incident Location and Facilities
9. Manageable Span of Control
10. Accountability
11. Information and Intelligence Management
12. Resource Management
13. Integrated Communications
14. Transfer of Command

During the 9/11 incident, the ICS was similarly found to be inadequate by itself. In particular, it was in need of a systematic overhaul with respect to the integration of responders from different jurisdictions and disciplines. The failures noted included a lack of accountability and of a planning process, poor communication, overloaded incident commanders, and no method for integrating interagency requirements. However, ICS remains a key feature that is integrated into the NIMS framework.

An executive order of former president George W. Bush in February 2003 set the stage for NIMS. The NIMS system consists of procedures for controlling personnel, facilities, equipment, and communications during planned events that go awry, natural disasters, and acts of terrorism.

The NIMS system, which embodies the 14 essential ICS features, provides a framework that is both flexible and integrative from a command-and-control structural viewpoint. It provides for the rapid assimilation of resources into a common modular, top-down organizational management structure. It imposes the concept of a manageable 'span of control,' which is limited to three to seven direct reports, with five being optimal. There are also defined chain of command, unity of command, and transfer of command processes with unequivocal duty assignments. The NIMS system allows for the provision of logistical and administrative support to operational staff. It also permits the use of common terminology and clear text without code words or jargon, which can cause confusion and errors based on misinterpretations of communications. There is also the assurance of an integrated communications system.

NIMS uses explicit guidance directed at cost-based effectiveness and the elimination or minimization of the duplication of effort. This occurs in concert with targeted resource deployments within an operational theater and resource utilization accountability. For this to occur efficiently, NIMS provides the basis for a process of management by objectives. This involves the creation of measurable, overarching objectives and assists in the development and issuing of plans, procedures, assignments, and protocols.

COL. Damon T. Arnold, M.D., M.P.H.

Creating an Incident Action Plan (IAP)

The creation of an IAP that coherently guides the operational and support activities for accomplishing the response objectives is essential. Only those positions critical to mission accomplishment are filled. Predesignated incident facilities and locations are also identified. NIMS runs in operational and support functions concordant with the Continuity of Operations Plan (COOP) for organizational planning, training, drills, and actual response purposes.

I have found that most often the critical infrastructure and key resource sectors involved in a disruption need to continue their usual, everyday functions. This is to ensure the provision of customary and essential community-based services during a disaster or disrupted event. It must be stressed that a NIMS-derived IAP and the institutional COOP share resources and have a heavy reliance upon each other, especially when resources are limited. Both the NIMS-derived IAP and the institutional COOP must be complementary and have as a central corollary that worker safety comes first.

It is essential that effective communication occurs for response efforts to be successful. All IAPs must have at least four basic elements: what needs to be done, who is responsible, how communication occurs, and what procedures to follow if worker injuries should occur. The IAP process helps in understanding the agency policy and direction, situational awareness assessments, and the establishment and selection of strategies to achieve objectives and goals. It also helps with tactical engagements. The After Action Report (AAR) is a necessary component of the evaluation process. It serves not only as a metric for prior performance but also as a tool and road map for the improvement of subsequent IAPs used to address similar situations in the future. Management by objectives is an approach used to communicate functional actions throughout the entire ICS organization.

The IAP, whether it is orally conveyed or written, must be completed for every incident. It must always be a written document for Hazmat situations and include objectives reflective of the overall strategy for incident management. This includes the identification of operational resources and assignments that provide additional direction.

Once again, this is just a brief overview of the NIMS system and some of the potential applications for its use. I strongly advise you to go online and complete the free training by visiting the federal FEMA website at www.fema.gov.

The concepts underlying NIMS fit exceedingly well in the fields of public health and occupational medicine as well as in the emergency response framework. Even during routine operational periods, NIMS principles can be applied to guide occupational and public health practices.

NIMS concepts lead to the creation of IAPs that can be applied readily to form effective implementation strategies directed at addressing the majority of issues encountered in the public health arena. Education, training, drills, and exercises are the keys to preparedness and to community-based health care. I advocate for the implementation of agency-wide and grantee IAP-based operational programs, not just for emergency situations but for general health intervention initiatives. They can also be designed in this setting to provide for grantee organizational development, education, training, drills, and exercises as a way to test their routine and emergency-based operational capabilities. This can be enacted prior to or upon grantee entry into a community.

The Emergency Operations Center (EOC) provides support and coordination, not management oversight, to on-scene responders and operations. It is important for the EOC operatives to know their roles and not to unnecessarily impede the activities of responders by attempting to control them. That is not the EOC's role. This fact is readily recognized by military personnel who engage in field operations but is sometimes forgotten in the civilian world.

Crossing the Silo Walls

In the literature, there has been much talk about the deconstruction of silo walls and the need to bridge these gaps through appropriate leadership interventions. At this juncture I recommend that you review *Chapter 3—The Relationship that Dwells Within*, especially the section titled *"Conflict Resolution and the Importance of Self Control,"* as well as *Chapter*

4—Words of Caution for Potential Interventionists, the section titled *"The Fallacies of Logic."* I feel these are important concepts to keep in mind when one is approaching issues within one's own—and across—silo walls. In *Chapter 3,* I stressed the importance of staying out of the CLAM'N (Coercion, Litigation, Arbitration, and Mediation). This is essential to a spirit of cooperation and collaboration directed at goal accomplishment. Negotiation is a much more effective tool for goal accomplishment when working with others.

In a community setting, there are many CIKR sectors present. These sometimes represent private-sector corporations, governmental public sector entities, or nonprofit philanthropic organizations. There are also faith-based institutions and many other nongovernmental, community-based organizations and advocacy groups.

As you cross the silo wall, be aware that there are several issues to address. Do it with a 'tool belt' containing familiar tools, such as action plans, drills, exercises, training concepts, and personal experiences. Your connectivity and mindfulness regarding the arenas you enter routinely or during a time of crisis are shaped by how well you have honed and fashioned these tools. If you have not prepared your tool belt in a disciplined way, it will not be available for use by you or your family, organization, or community when a specific response is needed to avert negative consequences arising from a disruptive situation.

Note that as you encounter others from a different silo, they may be wearing a different tool belt than yours. You may not readily recognize their tools and may tend to diminish their value because of your lack of familiarity and experience with them. You must therefore think beyond your own silo and intentionally connect with these persons in order to understand their viewpoint as well as how and why they must use their tools in various response situations. The synergy of such an association can be astounding when properly approached and applied.

Cross-Silo Connectivity and Operational Effectiveness

While in the military, I learned the importance of a chain of command structure. One must recognize and respect another person's position, authority, and influence. This must be mutual and binding on all parties involved. You must work collectively to guide activities, which are often based upon operational assumptions. To work from a common operational platform, there must be effective information sharing and communication as well as mutual support. There must also be social order and security for all individuals involved. You must be speaking the same language and understand the meaning of terms when they are used. Technical jargon is highly discouraged, as it can impede operational performance and lead to mistakes based on miscommunications, misinterpretations, and misconceptions. This is especially true when individuals are not familiar with or have no foundation in the discipline being discussed.

Be respectful of another person's opinions and perspectives. Whether you are leading or following at any moment, you must set a good example in your designated role. You must demonstrate positive qualities as a leader and a follower. You should provide the support above, across, and below your level at all times to ensure operational order, efficiency, and effectiveness. Demonstrating these qualities will encourage, inspire, and motivate the development of strong and effective subordinates who themselves will further galvanize your cross-silo connectivity and operational effectiveness. To do less puts you on the side of disruption and inflicts harm not only on operations but also on those you claim to be helping. You need to do a self-evaluation, or 'mirror test,' of what is effective and actually working for you in your various roles.

In addition, make sure you develop an awareness picture of what is going on and the scope of the situation. You must continuously note how this image changes as time progresses. You may also leverage resources across silos as you become more adept at this process. It is possible to carefully integrate missions and operations across silo walls as well. However, you must also be willing to respect another person's boundaries and the human dimensions of collaboration.

There are no perfect operations, but seek perfection in what you are attempting to accomplish as part of the team. Remember that time is on your side in preparedness training but an enemy during a disaster. Do not squander it during times of relative calm by being complacent when it comes to education, training, and drilling. These activities are important for creating an innate degree of self-confidence and personal resilience.

When responding to a crisis, remember to stay focused and avoid distractions. Work cooperatively, and focus on response effort goals and objectives. What the process yields as an outcome, and its value to those you are serving, will heavily depend upon what goes into the process. By participating in this way, you will discover new and better options for accomplishing the tasks at hand. Continuously build your levels of both competence and professional skills, and be aware of points when you are stepping outside your sphere of expertise and competence. When participating in this manner, you will develop a strengthened and broadened vantage point to respond from as a result of this cross-silo team approach. You will also establish trust with your peers, which is an invaluable asset.

In the next chapter, I will discuss the construction and development of a community-based kiosk system that addresses health from both prevention and monitoring perspectives.

Chapter 14

A Community-Based Medical Home Kiosk Model

I t remains obvious that disparities still exist with respect to information technology access during a period when such advancements are flourishing. This chapter focuses on a concept that may enhance the level of community engagement. This is especially true within impoverished community settings. All too often, the talents, abilities, skills, and genius of those that dwell within a community are extinguished by social injustices and the circumstances created by poverty. This externally imposed social marginalization and lack of resources conspires not only to deprive individuals but the entire community. In my work, I have encouraged the creation of functional models based upon information technology principles to bridge such a gap. In fact, the concept is quite simple, and multiple systems like this will be developed in this ever-accelerating computer—and information-driven age.

An Overview of the Kiosk System

To address community health care issues, I would like to present a relatively new concept in community engagement: the construction of a community-based kiosk system that presents health related information based upon best practice principles. It also contains health impact assessment metrics and analysis tools for in-depth analyses of intervention effectiveness.

Often it is difficult to specifically ascribe a definite causal relationship between an intervention strategy and an outcome. This is especially true in the case of very complex systems. The capability to record and transmit public data for epidemiological evaluation can potentially provide clues to the outcome on a population-based level. Despite the difficulty of establishing a direct causal link to a specific poor health outcome—what is important is the provision of resources—which most likely will reduce the risk for a poor outcome based on the use of best-practice principles.

I have chosen the topics of being overweight, obesity, and diabetes as examples to describe a proposed kiosk system intervention model. The intent is to create a sustainable platform from which to launch, orchestrate, and sustain a series of intervention strategies. These strategies are directed at providing educational materials, interactive exercises, and services in support of a community-based weight-control and obesity prevention program. The system also utilizes metrics that reflect the effectiveness of implemented strategies utilized within the kiosk system framework.

Although outside confounders may be difficult to control for, the implementation of effective best practice strategies can still be monitored. Both individual and collective weight, blood pressure, and blood sugar statuses can be recorded as well as compliance with a predetermined program.

Although weight management is the focus of this example, these principles can be applied to addictions to tobacco, alcohol, illicit drugs, and prescription medication. It can also be applied to oral health, safety, injury prevention, and a host of other public health concerns. In my view, injury prevention includes issues related to driving, patient safety, suicide, the workplace, and all forms of inflicted violence. Many times we silo these issues and develop unnecessarily complex and difficult problem-resolution constructs to address them. What we need now are simply, fundamental approaches to resolve these societal issues based upon a prevention-focused model.

Perhaps society as a whole with respect to its policies and practices can learn from an old medical saying: 'At first, do no harm.' It is decidedly more difficult to resolve an injury, illness, or disease process than it is to avoid its occurrence in the first place. This is why prevention is always the most prudent and logical path when addressing an agent that threatens an individual's or a community's health status.

Cultural Comprehension and Service

The kiosk model involves the establishment of two-way communication—that is, communication between the interventionist and the recipients of the intended education programs and services. This is provided via a bidirectional kiosk system. As noted previously in *Chapter 1—The Evolution of Human Adaptation, Perception, and Habituation,* one must first understand the culture from the viewpoint of the members of it who require services. Interceding without this understanding has caused countless intervention strategy failures, wasting valuable resources and causing actual harm. If you are not a part of the community, you cannot assume you know who they are and what they really need or want.

The kiosk belongs to the community you are attempting to assist. Your service interventions should not attempt to usurp the dignity, self-respect, and right to self-determination of community members. In approaching communities, you must not interfere with cultural practices in a 'take no prisoners' fashion.

You can only offer alternatives to norms that result in poor health outcomes. The decision to accept these alternatives remains with the community members themselves. This is essential for a truly effective and lasting cultural transformation.

The Kiosk System Initiative

The following is a summary and discussion of the strategic steps taken to guide the direction of this initiative. I pulled the sticky notes off the walls and avoided 'reinventing the wheel.' Attempts at reinvention can be very costly in terms of both money and time. I generally do not begin any discussions about how to address the cleanup of a chemical spill with attempts to reinvent the model for the sodium atom. We must learn to use available tools and to be creative with their use. This is not to say that inventive creativity is not needed. However, all too often individuals want to create their own tools, despite the existence and availability of a multiplicity of extremely effective ones.

Efforts must involve a coordinated partnership that brings all elements of the community and available resources together for a truly transformative process to occur. The resources must be utilized in a way that reduces unnecessary duplications and redundancies.

These concepts are reflected in the name I gave this project: Project Oneness: Restructuring the Wheel. Note that the term *restructuring* rather than *reinventing* is used. This emphasizes the point that many of the essential structural components already existing within the community can and must be blended with externally derived intervention resources. What is fundamentally required in this setting is organizational alignment and integration into a functional model rather than a reinvention of the components themselves.

People tend to want to make their own wheel, which I call 'the creator complex.' In these situations, which are all too common, it appears that the stroking of the ego is more important than the accomplishment of the task. This is extremely inefficient and costly. It can also block the fruition and implementation of truly creative and collaborative intervention strategies. Intervention efforts should also be directed at the creation of self-sustaining, self-sufficient models. Continued attempts at reinvention fail to support such modeling and indeed work against it.

We as a society have been relying on scientific and experiential discoveries from all parts of the world over millions of years. The Middle East, Africa, the Orient, and Europe are replete with a history of such discoveries. This has resulted in what the field of science is today. There is no need to reinvent the field of science.

A person may add to the field of science when possible. However, the utilization of the truly effective tools it has already yielded to address issues need to be implemented. Therefore, I chose to use the Centers for Disease Control (CDC) priority list to develop best-practice standards as the basis and starting point for the selection of areas requiring inclusion in the current planning process. In choosing to do this, I specifically avoided the temptation of reinvention.

The CDC lists the problems of obesity, tobacco abuse, and injury prevention as areas in need of national attention. The recommendations are for a national approach to addressing multiple health concerns with best-practice principles. The CDC has an excellent website (www. cdc.gov) of which you should take full advantage. There are many brilliant people within that institution, many of whom I know and admire. Their hard work has resulted in a readily available treasure chest of information and best practices on a variety of topics. Their work continues to pave the foundation for a healthier nation. Take advantage of this.

For illustrative purposes, I will focus on the issue of being overweight and some of its resultant health consequences. Both the premorbid and the morbidity-associated consequences of being overweight, yield data which can serve as metrics for the evaluation of an individual's health status. Unfortunately, we as a society have chosen to rely on the diagnosis and treatment of diseases rather than on their prevention.

The kiosk system model I have developed monitors body mass index (BMI), blood pressure, and blood sugar levels. It also educates individuals on the need for compliance with recommended exercise and nutritional practices. Required, routine screenings for ongoing health care, such as vision and foot care for those with diabetes, are also emphasized. Each individual using the kiosk benefits from personal information and educational experiences. And the public aggregate data can define population trends in groups utilizing the kiosk, which is tied to a specific intervention strategy. The purpose is to measure and determine whether the methods employed are truly effective as a population-based intervention strategy.

The focus is on the creation of a metrically driven, best-practice intervention model that strategically targets and eliminates the causal factors for obesity—while providing incentives for programmatic compliance and yielding kiosk-derived performance metrics. This prototypical model directed at weight reduction can also be applied to numerous other unhealthy behaviors that result in avoidable pain, suffering, and premature death. Once enacted, best-practice models can be measured by such a mechanism with predetermined parameters for gauging their effectiveness. This will involve the input of the community serviced, which will have ownership of the community-based kiosk. Such a system is best supported by the private business infrastructure, not the public sector.

Most political and public entities battle with equity based upon one or another social determinant of health. Despite this, I feel what is truly needed for a community-based, health-centered cultural transformation to take place is what I call '*infrastructure equity.*' This involves the realization of risk reductions in relation to the occurrence of pain, suffering, and premature death—through the development of critical infrastructure and key resource sectors that support healthy lifestyles.

This includes good schools, transportation services, grocery stores, and other adequately constructed infrastructure and resource sectors. By investing correctly in these sectors, a self-sustainable, healthy community infrastructure can be achieved and poor outcomes averted. It will also inculcate within the community members a sense of self-determination and self-worth.

Interventionists should recognize and find points of alignment with the objectives of their State Health Improvement Plan (SHIP) framework. For example, as the director of public health for my state of Illinois, I designed the SHIP framework in the form of a public-private partnership model, with various platforms to address specific health care issues. It allows agencies such as those involved with human services, education, and economics to participate fully in the process. Private industries, advocacy groups, and community members from the areas to be serviced should be heavily involved in this process.

No one individual or organization owns any of the SHIP framework platforms. This is due to the fact that no one individual or organization has the capacity, resources, or insight to service everyone within a community, much less the state. In fact, any attempt to form splinter groups or consensus groups within the body of platform members undermines the trust of the other individuals involved in the process. This is a movement away from true collaboration. It will obstruct progress and poison the entire initiative. I feel that such actions actually aid and abet, and thereby become complicit in, the appearance of pain, suffering, and premature death within communities in need of supportive services.

This kiosk approach allows for a focused, best-practices-based, integrated, and cohesive conceptual approach to public health concerns. Again, the focus here is on weight control, obesity, and diabetes. The kiosk system provides education and guidance concerning proper nutrition, exercise, and medical system care integration to community members. This is coupled with a scientifically-based, metrics-driven, analytical component that yields a Health Impact Assessment (HAI) statement that can be utilized for the evaluation of an intervention strategy.

As explained earlier, however, there is still a need to develop a contextual implementation strategy for any intervention methodology. This implies a need to provide a certain degree of flexibility in its application with respect to the community member's viewpoints. All too often there is a tendency for those who are unenlightened and who lack vision to reject the mechanisms by which a community chooses to implement its intervention strategies. A true intellectual and scientist would never do this. Pseudo-scientists, and those with little if any knowledge or training in such concerns, should not tread here. I have witnessed many projects being flatly rejected by the powers that be, only to be implemented through community-based persistence that yielded amazing results.

The involved community members must clearly understand, trust in, and accept what you are bringing to them. They must also feel a degree of ownership of and sense of control over the progressive integration of the intervention strategy.

I also highly recommend, at a minimum, the pursuit of training in the National Incident Management System (NIMS) 100, 200, 700, and 800 courses on the FEMA website (www.fema.gov). This should be followed by the didactic, as face-to-face-classroom training in the NIMS 300 and 400 level courses. It is especially important for those in any discipline within the public health arena where they will serve in a senior management position or on an intervention response team. This form of training can dramatically increase your operational efficiency and effectiveness during a response to a man-made or natural disaster but also has implications for routine workplace activities.

There is a tendency to categorize H1N1 as an emergency while not classifying the spread of HIV infections or the growing prevalence of obesity in the same way. Not only does the medical field and society as a whole need to modernize its thinking on this point, but an effort to apply the principles underlying NIMS to such issues should be made as well.

Cross-silo, meta-leadership concepts can also be applied in this context. This crosses silo walls to gain the benefits from positive synergisms that arise through collaboration. As I noted earlier, NIMS and ICS organizational and business principles can be extended effectively to all public health problems, including such issues as weight control, diabetes, and obesity. They can guide the planning and construction of community-based operational intervention (incident) action plans.

A complete legislative review to determine where various rules, laws, and regulations stand with respect to obesity and diabetes is also helpful. They should be reviewed for content, intent, and congruence with respect to the intended interventional approaches to be utilized. A grantee selection, tracking, monitoring, and evaluation system should also be in place for the coordination of the various entities involved but also for the implementation of best practice-based performance metrics. This is essential, as the grantee deliverables generated by such a process must be aligned with the parameters used to measure the effectiveness of the best practice-based prevention strategy—that is, from the perspective of the prevention strategy being implemented within the context of the community setting.

A Practical, Real-World Application of the Kiosk System

Currently two-thirds of adults and one-third of children in the United States are overweight, according to recent national reports on obesity. This threatens not only our national but also our domestic security interests. If we are unable, due to the lack of physical readiness of potential recruits, to raise a military, firefighting, policing, labor, or medical responder workforce, both national and domestic security are fundamentally at risk. This provides fertile ground for the use of a kiosk-based system as described below.

Concerns Regarding the Alarming Rate of Obesity

In 1985 the World Health Organization (WHO) noted that there were about 30 million people living with diabetes globally. Currently this number is more than 197 million. A projection notes that this number will increase to 300 million by the year 2025—a tenfold increase worldwide since 1985. There will also be a rise in the global population from the current approximately seven to an estimated 10 to 12 billion people. If this trend continues, we will never be able to provide the resources or services required to meet the medical needs arising from obesity and a global population explosion. This is especially true in a society bent on approaching health with a medical system based on a treatment model. If we do not invest heavily in prevention starting now, we will have sealed our population-based poor health outcome fate.

In the United States, diabetes is the leading cause of nontraumatic lower-limb amputations, blindness in adults 20 to 74 years of age, and kidney failure leading to the need for renal dialysis. In addition, 65 to 70 percent of those with diabetes die from heart disease and stroke due to vascular complications. It should be noted that the resulting vascular disease is the pathway to death for a majority of those who have poorly controlled diabetes.

If not treated, diabetes can cause life-threatening events, such as high blood sugar levels resulting in comas, heart attacks, and strokes. Obesity is defined as being 30 percent or more over one's ideal body weight based on the body mass index (BMI). However, one can be moderately or grossly overweight without meeting the definition for obesity and still be at risk for health related problems.

Public Law 111-148, HR3590—The Patient Protection and Affordable Care Act—was signed into law by President Barack Obama on March 23, 2010. Title IV of President this act is entitled "Prevention of Chronic Disease and Improving Public Health." This act is a valuable resource when aligning the framework of this concept with the directives issued by the federal government. The act clearly notes a need for strengthening wellness and prevention efforts to address the health issues confronting our nation. This was a visionary stroke of genius on the part of President Obama.

Following is list of the titles of the Patient Protection and Affordable Care Act is provided:

Title I: Quality, Affordable Health Care for All Americans
Title II: The Role of Public Programs
Title III: Improving the Quality and Efficiency of Health Care
Title IV: Prevention of Chronic Disease and Improving Public Health
Title V: Health Care Work Force
Title VI: Transparency and Program Integrity
Title VII: Improving Access to Innovative Medical Therapies
Title VIII: Community Living Assistance Services and Support (CLASS) Act
Title IX: Revenue Provisions
Title X: Reauthorization of the Indian Health Care Improvement Act

Both nutrition and exercise are essential components of any intervention plan attempting to combat the problem of obesity. This fact was astutely noted to be a major target issue for the American public by First Lady Michelle Obama with her 'Let's Move' campaign. We must increase consumption of fruits, vegetables, and whole grains as part of our daily diet. At the same time, avoidance of products containing saturated fat, cholesterol, and salt as well as high-calorie, sugar-sweetened food must be adhered to.

The Influence of Evolution

I have theorized that as humans developed in natural settings, the drive to obtain a meal was a daunting task. This hunt for food often occurred in austere environments that provided scarce nutritional resources. This set the stage for a cycle of triumphs and defeats in the quest for nutritious food and the very survival of the individual. As a result, I speculate that we developed a taste for and a drive to obtain certain substances as part of our innate survival skills. This included fat, which is high in calories; salt, which is scarce in inland environments; and sugar, which provides an immediate source of biologically available energy.

These sources of nutrition in an austere environment provide a survival advantage when consumed. They are not usually readily available, and energy must be expended in the hunting and collecting process to obtain these nutritional resources. In nature, the balance between the energy expended and the energy obtained in this hunting effort must be beneficial and weighted in the direction of survival.

Although these higher calorie nutritional sources in the past were the trophies of a successful hunt, in the modern world we do not have to hunt for food every day. These food sources are, all too often, readily available. Both sugar and salt have historically been, and still are, used to preserve foods. Because of our instinctual drive to seek them out and their value as natural preservatives, manufacturers have chosen to use them in food products. Sugar and salt extend the shelf life of food products and prevent the need for refrigeration, which has an associated cost.

These sweet and salty food items are more attractive and marketable to us, the consumers. They are more palatable and potentially addictive to us because of our instinctual, biological drive to seek them out. We are, however, now consuming harmful amounts of readily available fats, sugars, salt, and other additives as part of our daily diet, with dire consequences flowing from these decisions.

COL. Damon T. Arnold, M.D., M.P.H.

An Alternative Approach to Satiate Our Natural Drives

Alternative practices can be employed to overcome this tendency toward consuming products that are harmful to our health. For example, water is better for satiating one's thirst than a high-calorie beverage. Breastfeeding for infants is also strongly encouraged, because it has been noted to decrease the risk for obesity and a myriad of other health-related problems in children.

A sedentary lifestyle should be avoided; physical exercise should become a routine part of daily life. In some impoverished areas, residents cite safety concerns as a reason for not exercising. The movement toward the construction of safer infrastructures for such communities is ideal. Attempts should also be made to create safe zones in existing community structures—while we wait for construction and resource allocations to become available. This may take decades to occur in the current fiscal climate. In the context of these fiscally challenging times, the procurement of the capital and resources required for such infrastructure construction is difficult. This is especially true in impoverished communities that have been ignored. We do not have the luxury of being able to wait decades before implementing a prevention plan that works.

As noted, obesity is increasing on a global scale. It is estimated that approximately one-third of children are overweight. For the first time in recorded history, children are being diagnosed with type 2 diabetes—and at an alarming rate. According to the CDC, these children will for the first time in history have a shorter life span than their parents. I strongly maintain that we cannot afford the prospect of turning our classrooms into health treatment centers. This has staggering implications for the educational system. It actually threatens not only educational activities but also the production of adequately educated individuals to compete in the global economy.

The percentage for adults over the age of 20 years old who are considered by clinical standards to be overweight is approximately 66. Also, over half of these individuals fit the criteria for being classified as being obese, having a BMI of 30 to 40 percent higher than recommended. Further, almost five percent of those who are overweight can be classified as having extreme obesity—having a BMI of 40 percent or more.

The presence of obesity involves a host of factors, including polygenic and less commonly monogenic genetic patterns. However, in the overwhelming majority of cases, the lack of exercise and poor nutrition underpin the onset of obesity and poor health. Therefore, prevention efforts largely focus on this balance between exercise and nutrition—the cornerstones of weight management. On a physiological basis, obesity results from an imbalance between energy intake (input) and energy expenditure (output). In Eastern medicine terms, this can be visualized as an imbalance between yang (energy) and yin (matter), creating a tendency toward mass and matter accumulation.

The behavioral aspects of this tendency toward unhealthy weight gains must also be addressed. Attention must be paid to what motivations and drives are operative and lead people to participate in unhealthy practices in the first place. These unhealthy practices cycles must be addressed and replaced by healthy lifestyle practices. Such healthy practices must take into account the psychological and emotional underpinnings of the individual being serviced.

Obesity has been tied to risk factors such as the chronic ingestion of excess calories, a poor-quality diet, a sedentary lifestyle, and even sleep deprivation. I strongly feel that the advent of depression and overeating as a psychosocial coping mechanism must receive greater attention. Truly, we must come out of the dark ages with respect to the treatment of mental health and behavioral issues in this country.

To calculate BMI, follow these steps:

1. Multiply your height in inches by your height in inches (height in inches squared)
2. Divide your weight in pounds by the result obtained in step 1
3. Multiply your result from step 2 by 703 to obtain your BMI

For example, if a person weighs 180 pounds and is 5'9" tall then the BMI may be calculated as:

153

$$BMI = \frac{180 \text{ pounds}}{(69 \text{ inches}) (69 \text{ inches})} \times 703 = 26.6$$

This result is your Body Mass Index (BMI). It represents your relative excess of adipose (fatty) tissue mass. It can be compared to the table below for classification purposes.

< 25 "Normal"
> 25 Overweight
> 30 Obesity: [Class I (BMI 30—35)] and [Class II (BMI 35—40)]
> 40 Extreme Obesity: [Class III (BMI > 40)]

The BMI of 25 is the borderline for "normal." The term *normal* is in quotation marks as there are experts who feel that even this number is set too high for a healthy weight. The key here is that obesity most often results from a high caloric intake and a sedentary lifestyle, lacking in a significant amount of physical exercise. Clearly, this is inconsistent with the outcome of a healthy lifetime.

It has been well established in scientific literature that obesity, a sedentary lifestyle, and poor nutrition are risk factors for numerous chronic diseases. Among others, these medical conditions include type 2 diabetes, hypertension, hyperlipidemia, stroke, cardiovascular disease, congestive heart failure, obstructive sleep apnea, hepatitis, degenerative arthritis, and gallstones.

The development of diabetes as a result of being overweight occurs when the nutritional and exercise components of an individual are out of balance. This occurs when the behaviors of an individual move them in a direction that leads to a positive weight gain beyond established body-weight recommendations. When this occurs, the pancreas, where insulin is produced, is unable to keep up with the increased demand for insulin production.

The hormone insulin helps the sugar glucose to enter cells for use as a fuel source or for its storage in cells for future use. When not enough insulin is produced by the body, this results in high blood sugar levels. Since glucose cannot enter the cells due to a lack of the required amount of insulin, the glucose remains in the blood.

This results in increased thirst and the drinking of water as the body tries to eliminate sugar by washing it out. This causes the person to urinate excessively in an attempt to rid his or her body of the excessive amount of sugar in the blood. The loss of water with the sugar can lead to dehydration. The nervous system, which does not require insulin for sugar to enter nerve cells, is particularly vulnerable to the damaging effects of high sugar levels. Dizziness, confusion, and even a coma can result when high sugar levels are present and go unchecked.

The health consequences arising from diabetes, therefore, require the use of medical interventions aimed at maintaining normal blood sugar levels. This is aimed at palliating the physiological and pathological consequences arising from the diabetes disease process. The presence of obesity can also directly exacerbate other coexisting conditions, such as heart disease, hypertension, asthma, and arthritis. Cigarette smoking is an independent risk factor for the development of comorbidities in a person with diabetes and accelerates the progression of vascular disease. Vascular disease is the common pathway leading to death in most cases of diabetes.

The prevention of diseases associated with being overweight involves a focus on nutrition and exercise. However, behavioral and infrastructure food access issues must be addressed as well. Treatment-centric models focus on specific disease states and the typical palliative therapies and procedures aimed at controlling the disease progression and complications. Many curative methods, such as islet cell transplants and the duodenal switch procedure, are currently experimental but have been yielding very encouraging results. In addition to adequate medical follow-up and treatment for those with diabetes, specific community-based intervention strategies aimed at prevention can be included in a therapeutic regimen. A prevention-centric focus should be extended throughout the treatment spectrum, regardless of the stage of the injury, illness, or disease.

The establishment and use of farmer's markets, food delivery services, exercise regimens, and education-centered service programs can greatly assist this process. This is especially helpful in food deserts where poor access to nutritious foods exists and few resources are present.

Food deserts may occur in inner-city or rural environments as well as in sports stadiums. A food desert is an issue of food choice access, not just location. It is a matter of the quality of the choices that exist at a location where food is available for consumption. A similar analogy can be made with respect to medical care institutions. It is not just an issue of the existence of an access point, but the quality of the services that are provided there as well.

A Prevention-Based Community Kiosk Model

The prevention-based model that I have developed involves the creation and placement of a fixed, community-based medical kiosk system in nongovernmental organization sites. I have chosen faith-based institutions and public locations for some of the planned pilot sites. This is due to the presence and leveraging of several cultural and inherent trust factors encountered within these community-based locations. I have the opinion that community members must feel a sense of ownership of the actual physical hardware of the kiosk site for it to have the desired impact. In fact, it should be viewed as a tool that enables individuals to take care of themselves, while conferring some degree of user control over the process. Community members should feel empowered to take care of themselves as a result of participation in this process.

A kiosk prototype is presented in Figure 8 on the next page.

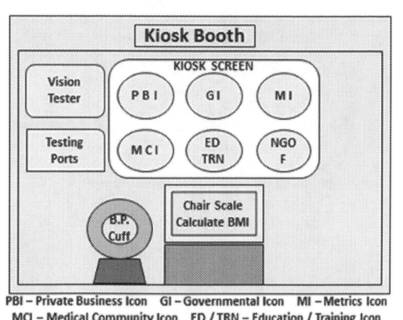

Figure 8. Diagram of Kiosk Model

This concept can also be designed for intercommunication with home computers and telemedicine systems as well as cellular phone messaging and texting, Twitter, or other communication formats. Some of the benefits of a community-based medical home kiosk in faith-based institutions are as follows:

1. Faith-based leaders have a spiritually based approach that includes compassion, ethics, a sense of morality, and an orientation toward the situational needs of their followers. This occurs on a mental, emotional, and physical as well as a spiritual level. They also engender a high degree of trust from their followers, which is essential for compliance with an intervention strategy.

2. There is often a long term relationship between followers and their faith-based institutional leaders. This often includes

family groups over several generations. This provides for the long-term and relatively well-defined periodic participation and follow-up of intervention program participants at the faith-based institution. Longitudinal, family-focused follow-up is also possible in this setting.

3. The kiosk system can be initially placed in faith-based institutions with 10,000 members or more. This will provide for a better statistical and epidemiology-based analysis of the de-identified data generated. A metrically based analysis of intervention effectiveness can also be obtained in this setting. This does not imply, however, that the kiosk services would be of any less benefit at faith-based institutions with smaller membership numbers.

4. Faith-based leaders can provide guidance as well as create follower support group activities, sermons, and other supportive services. These can be organized and directed at addressing the issues related to obesity and other health topics.

5. Larger faith-based institutions are also more likely to have doctors, nurses, paramedics, emergency medical technicians, and volunteer personnel as a part of their membership pool. These individuals, if they are so inclined, can serve both in the deployment of the kiosk system and act as sources of medical expertise. Psychiatrists, psychologists, and social workers usually are associated with faith-based institutions as well, and can be an indispensable aid in the process.

6. Faith-based leaders can choose to use this intervention method continuously throughout the week or offer access to the kiosk during planned activities. It can be used for focus groups of members, indigent populations, and other collective group activities. The establishment of community health teams to support this faith-based, member-centered medical initiative can also be of great benefit to all involved.

Some of the features of a fixed, community-based medical home kiosk:

1. The kiosk's structural design consists of a booth with a privacy compartment containing a chair that can measure an individual's weight and a mounted, individualized touch computer screen. There are several testing portals and instructional icons as well. This is illustrated in Figure 8 above.

2. The computer screen organization and dashboard design consist of an avatar guidance system and icons dedicated to key stakeholder information, including data inputs, participant learning activities, and assessment tools. The icons were created to cover the following topical areas of concern:

    *   *Government (public) icon:* The governmental icon can have links to credible federal, state, local, and tribal information and supportive resources concerned with addressing the issue of obesity and other health-related matters. It can organize infrastructure issues into an intelligible framework for use by kiosk end-users. The aim is to deal with the complexities of various services within the critical infrastructure and key resource sectors within community-based settings in such a way as to make them user-friendly and accessible.

    *   *Business (private) icon:* The business section includes pharmacies, clothing stores, fitness clubs, farmer's markets, insurance companies, and other businesses. These entities can provide discounts and other incentives for utilization and for progress made in losing weight. Clothing stores may choose to participate and provide discounts to those who lose weight and have a significant clothing size change. For example, a clothing store may offer the person who drops two garment sizes 50 percent off on clothing up to a 500 dollar value. This incentive can serve as a reward for losing the weight and also as a marketing tool for the clothing store. Additionally, this may partially remove an often-cited obstacle to losing weight: having to buy new clothing.

The private business partners can be charged a nominal user fee for participation and advertising on the kiosk dashboard to help defray the costs of kiosk operations, support, and maintenance. Such a relationship supports the requisite business infrastructure for a self-sustaining intervention strategy. This may also allow private businesses to make lasting customer-based relationships with those they assist in this process of becoming healthier.

- *Medical community icon:* The medical community at large, or locally, may provide pertinent information about health concerns. This results in a strengthened relationship between the community members and their health care providers. This can also provide a platform for the implementation of a telemedicine network. Also, local health departments or a federally qualified health center (FQHCs) may be able to use this to communicate with patients for monitoring purposes.

The passage of the Affordable Care Act also provides the opportunity for providers to save time and make a greater impact on their patients' health. Providers are now confronting an insurance pool projected to contain more than double the number of participants as previously encountered. If the provider's office has double the patient load and no change in office support, the contact time per patient will likely be cut in half. A typical 15-minute visit will now be 7.5-minutes in duration. Such a situation may be addressed by the provider utilizing the kiosk system. For instance, the provider can make video recordings for patient education on basic topics such as high blood pressure, diabetes, and other medical concerns.

The patient will see the provider explaining the topic and will have a basic understanding of his or her medical issues during the visit. This will allow the patient to ask informed health-related questions. The provider will not have to waste valuable time going over all the basic principles explained in the video and can focus on more important issues for the patient to consider. As a result, time will be saved and the quality of the visit will improve. These recordings can also be made available for use on the kiosk, at home, or in the medical office waiting area. A Poison Control Center may choose to provide information on home safety issues when dealing with food preservation, preparation, and storage as well as household chemicals including those underneath the kitchen sink.

This can be developed in parallel with current ongoing efforts directed at the creation of health information exchanges. In the future, the kiosk may also become a secured location for the collection and viewing or downloading of an individual's medical information and records.

- *Metrics icon:* The metrics section can establish a baseline and follow the subsequent progress of any individual or the de-identified data of a group of individuals to monitor progress. The provision of feedback on their progress along with suggested steps for further progress can be made available in the form of a printed or downloadable document. Each participant is provided with a personalized kiosk access number specific to him or her. A card or touch-screen entry system can be used for the initial encounter. The person is then instructed to enter a password into the kiosk system. This allows the individual to access to his or her personal information with a pass code known only to that person. Personal progress reports will not contain any personal identification information, such as a full name or Social Security number. A code word or nickname can be assigned to the account for personal security. This also sets the stage for the collection of de-identified data over a long period.

The data can then be analyzed and drilled down to the individual, the hosting institution, or the established network sites in the aggregate. The progress of an individual can be tracked as he or she follows one or more intervention method. Hemoglobin A1C, BMI, and blood sugars can be followed to determine the progress of an individual or a specified group of individuals.

A site may also wish to include the ability to take blood pressure or other diagnostic measurements. The kiosk is able to measure and enter data such as weight, height, blood pressure, and blood sugar level. The results can be accessed when the individual enters his or her password into the protected site. The individual will never need to enter personal information that identifies who he or she is. The de-identified data results are fed directly into the metrics icon.

De-identified information and data can be collected and conveyed to a central computer, where it can be analyzed by statisticians and epidemiologists. The results of this de-identified data analysis can then be utilized to determine the effectiveness of a specific intervention strategy. Information generated in this way can also serve in helping to redesign, or design new, future intervention methodologies. It can be shared and utilized by all partners, including the oversight health-based organizations, policymakers, and most importantly, the affected community members themselves.

This plan can also be modified and the individual or group can provide feedback as to how the process is or is not working for them. For example, in an unsafe food desert area, a dietary plan that includes the weekly provision of farmer's market fruits and vegetables can be established. It can then be linked with an athletic center exercise program for an individual or group, or with the LINK card and WIC programs. This can then be followed for both programmatic compliance and effectiveness.

The participant has the ability to provide feedback on the implementation of intervention programs and can be asked whether adjustments would help in their particular case for compliance purposes. This process may also lead to the discovery and development of new best-practice approaches for use within the community setting, while allowing intervention flexibility and adaptability at the local level. It will ensure that all levels—from federal to local to tribal, and back to federal—will be involved in the process and receive the requisite data on which to make future intervention plans and decisions.

- *Nongovernmental organizations icon:* The nongovernmental icon can include entities such as grantee and non-profit organizations and volunteers. These organizations may be involved with the provision of on-site or off-site services. For example, volunteer organizations can also use a trained adult or youth volunteer to help technology-challenged individuals digitize their personal documents, information, and family photographs onto a CD or DVD format. This would be very useful for senior community members should they experience an emergency or disaster situation.

- *Training icon:* The training icon can be used to instruct individual users on personal medical matters. It can also be used for educational instruction leading to a volunteer training certificate program. Faith-based leaders can also include health sermons and talks as part of their instructional practices. They can serve as guides, directing their followers to healthier lifestyles and encouraging them to seek medical care for a better health outcome.

Local providers can also create instructional videos and visit checklists for the participants to take to their health care appointments. Instructional videos can also be used to prepare and educate individuals with information that a provider does not have time to explain during the standard office visit. This can also serve as the prerequisite for a deeper, more focused conversation concerning the individual's medical care.

This may also be used to lay the foundation for inspiring members of faith-based institutions to pursue careers in health care. This is especially true for careers in which projections reflect the need for an increased health worker pool. This is consistent with Title V of President Obama's Patient Protection and Affordable Care Act regarding workforce development.

I envisioned and contributed to the development of a kiosk system that incorporates many of these components. Additional icons can be created to cover a wide range of medical needs and services oriented toward improving the general public health. There are also several models already in existence of kiosks covering a range of issues pertinent to the needs of the general public. The field of medical informatics is rapidly progressing. This should become easier to implement in the very near future, as technologies become more advanced, accessible, and cost-effective. It must be borne in mind that this is only one potential intervention strategy.

A word of caution is required at this point. With computer-based technology, one must never forget that the user of the system is still a living, breathing human being. We must respect moral, ethical, privacy, and legal boundaries whenever we attempt to implement such a kiosk model system. Hopefully, we will never forget this fact as we move further into an information-driven technological age. An explanation of these various issues is beyond the scope of this book. It requires a thoughtful approach and the guidance of those with expertise in these various areas of concern, involving several disciplines. Before constructing and implementing such a system, it is very important, and wise, to seek this form of guidance.

In the next chapter, I will discuss the creation of a public health fusion center concept. This involves the discussion of an approach called SMART DOC (Strategic Management and Resource Technology Department Operations Center). This serves as a center for organizational planning, management, operational control, and training.

Chapter 15

The Need for a Public Health Fusion Center

SMART DOC

Often there is expressed the need for a tool that would provide a level of awareness of community needs and activities from a population-based vantage point. I devised the concept of the Strategic Management and Resource Technology—Department Operations Center (SMART DOC) conceptual model to address this need. It is directed at the construction of a continuously operating, public health-focused fusion center. The salient features of SMART DOC are its ability to operate continuously and provide situational awareness reports regarding population-based health concerns. It is essentially a continuously operating, public health-focused fusion center. I have listed an article in the references that I wrote in the fall of 2007 for the Journal of Homeland Security regarding the need for public health fusion centers.

Population-based perspectives are ever more important in setting social policies and practices at every level of society. This involves arenas dealing with complex issues such as the fiscal management of various health care models, homeland security strategies, and routine public health practices. However, this goes further to include health-related inputs into entities such as the criminal justice, educational, commerce, and economic systems.

The existence of a public health fusion center is especially needed in our current environmental and social climate. Response times should be shortened, focused, and more appropriately applied to event and incident management situations as a result of applying the information derived from such fusion centers. To date, not much has been done to address this need in an organized fashion. This effort requires the partial deconstruction of existing silos, not only on an agency-centric organizational level but also on the basis of fundamental legislative policy as well.

I have transformed the concept of a focused fusion center with a law enforcement-focus to one with a public health focus at its core. This concept provides a platform for the provision of timely and actionable health information for the betterment of a community's health status. The concept allows for consistency with and the inclusion of ICS and NIMS principles. This approach also parallel's the Department of Homeland Security's Strategic Plan (2008). This plan calls for using an all-hazards approach, capitalizing on emerging technologies, and working as an integrated response team.

The purpose of this fusion center is to make further progress toward the goal of public health in combating morbidity and premature mortality in an organized fashion—that is, providing a greater degree of health and safety for the welfare of the community as a whole in an increasingly complex environment.

This fusion center addresses the mitigation of health-related risk factors. It offers a higher level of protection through the intelligent use of information and data generated within the public health system. This information and data will be shared with partner organizations in the public sector to increase societal stability and resilience at the community level. It will also provide the basis for interactions with partners within private medical provider businesses and community-based organizations.

This fusion center will anticipate, monitor, detect, identify, and provide data on public health concerns related to acute and chronic medical and baseline conditions. It will also cover terrorist, man-made, and natural events and incidents. The public health fusion center also informs, educates, and empowers the community members with respect to health-related issues. Community members must participate in the mitigation and potential elimination of health-related risk factors. They must also be involved in discussions involving community-based medical care. Regulations, laws, and policies that protect the health of the community members must be successfully applied and appropriately enforced.

Community interventions must be evaluated from the viewpoints of effectiveness, accessibility, and quality. New insights, innovative solutions, and community engagement must be components of the fusion center plan. However, even as we respond to incidents, we cannot ignore the ever-present forms of acute and chronic disease during a natural or man-made incident. The prevention and treatment of the morbidity and mortality that arises from harmful incidents must be recognized and either eliminated or mitigated. This process is essential in order to reduce the societal impact of any potential or evolving health concern or incident.

Both short—and long-term recovery efforts must include plans for the management of acute and chronic illnesses, injuries, and diseases. This also includes mortuary services for fatalities that occur. The timeline for public health responses can last from hours to years after the occurrence of an incident. Public health workers truly never leave the field. The intent is to have situational awareness, structured organizational processes, and an integrated view of the event or incident at hand.

The SMART DOC concept utilizes a management dashboard, geo-coding, and graphical displays to improve the interpretation and comprehension of information and data. Within this system a general awareness of established and important public health parameters is generated. It has similarities to the law enforcement-focused fusion center, which tends to concentrate on criminal activities, incident sites, and events. A person suspected of engaging in criminal activity can experience several possible outcomes, including criminal prosecution – if convicted, sentencing can range from efforts at preventing recidivism to life or short-term imprisonment with or without parole and on to the death penalty.

What I propose here is that the same organizational matrix that underlies the criminal justice model be applied to the medical and public health models. The ability to explain the relationship between the various criminal activities and criminal justice system outcomes can be used to relate various health care practices, behaviors, and outcomes. The outcomes related to activities that arise from poor health practices and behaviors can be analogized to criminal justice system outcomes. Rather than the death penalty in the criminal justice system, there may be a limb amputation or death that occurs as a correlate in the medical system. Instead of life or limited sentencing in the criminal justice system, short-term or lifelong therapy for pneumonia or diabetes, respectively, may be indicated in the medical system. The need to prevent recidivism in the criminal justice system is similar to the need to prevent recurrent injuries, illnesses, and diseases in the medical system with counseling and education.

These comparisons are made to illustrate the fact that both the criminal justice and the medical systems have an array of outcomes with similar endpoints. The medical and public health systems outcomes, and the critical infrastructure and key resource sector features that underlie them, can be inserted into a fusion center matrix—that is, one similar to that of the criminal justice system fusion center matrix.

The matrix is structured to yield an explanation of how these elements are interrelated. It reveals relationships that are not as obvious upon superficial examination of the independent parts. It also reveals potential underlying collaborations and conflicts with associated synergisms and antagonisms, respectively. This brings to light the issues raised earlier in the book—that is, the integration of the energy-matter spectrum approach, which identifies all the agents relevant to a specific health care issue.

Why Is There a Need for a Medical and Public Health Fusion Center?

The need for a public health fusion center is based upon the varied, vacillating, and increasingly complex nature of public health's roles and responsibilities within the communities it serves. Public health responders remain involved in an emergency long after other response elements have withdrawn their services through demobilization and dismissal.

Public health must address both the short-term and long-term impacts of any incident or disrupted event. It is also charged with monitoring chronic disease conditions that may subsequently arise as a result of these disruptive situations. Such conditions may have been exacerbated, or even caused, by the incident or event that goes awry.

Public health also needs to track and attempt to mitigate the incidence of infectious diseases or the emergence of other agents that may lag behind the initial disruptive occurrence. For example, the threat of West Nile Virus transmission may be increased if the factors supporting the breeding of vector mosquitoes, which spread the virus, increase during a season. By understanding this relationship one can preplace vector mitigation agents such as insecticides and larvacide agents in a region that is projected to be increasingly favorable for vector breading. This can minimize or eliminate an infestation of biting insects that threatens to erode operational efficiency in the field environment.

A public health fusion center can greatly increase situational awareness for public health workers and other responders present in the environment. The fusion center can also track employee activities and the provision of support services. It can also be crafted to integrate and handle the all-important balancing of the Continuity of Operations Plan (COOP) with the response effort needs at hand.

Common Threads

Common threads span the public health system as it passes through the federal, state, local, and tribal levels. These threads can be envisioned as existing within a common conduit that crosses through each level from the federal to the community setting. This relationship is depicted in Figure 6 in *Chapter 9—A Social Disruption Model for Interventionists.* The conduit passes through the environmental, monitoring, incident, primary treatment, secondary treatment, and community home sites.

Within the realm of the public health system, this can include such components as the following:

1. Communication (internal and external)
2. Subject matter expertise
3. Planning
4. Policy
5. Education, training, certifications, and licensures
6. Exercises and drills
7. Intelligence and analysis
8. Security
9. Legal
10. Safety
11. Resources (equipment, personnel, and strategic/operational partners)
12. Intervention and response triggers (tribal, local, state, and federal)
13. Time scale for various operational periods
14. Performance metrics
15. Response capacities and capabilities (minimum and maximum)

The field of public health has often been inaccurately viewed as what I refer to as a 'Pasteurian' construct—that is, bound solely to microbiological concepts related to bacteria and viruses. In actuality, public health covers a vast spectrum of issues from quantum and particle physics to chemistry to biology, including the food chains. It covers every energy-matter relationship from particle physics to the food chain.

With respect to disaster response and preparedness issues, public health also involves considerations surrounding terrorist acts as well as geophysical and weather-related phenomena. These phenomena are all transitional energy-matter relationships that are guided by the central axis of the laws of physics. It is of fundamental importance to approach these phenomena in a rational, scientific fashion. However, it is also important to always remember that they are modified by extrinsic as well as intrinsic human behavioral factors. This includes the available

CIKR sector resources and the relative level of preparedness of the involved community members. This may vary greatly from community to community and as an individual or group move from the natural to the home or work environment.

Our health care infrastructure is comprised of public health departments, hospitals, federally qualified health care centers, various outpatient procedure centers, clinics, and private practices. These entities collect, analyze, and disseminate medical information and intelligence routinely. However, there is a strong need for various components of the medical community to address health concerns in a unified, well-integrated, and efficient fashion. This system must also favor prevention over treatment. Treatment is still important, but a lost opportunity for prevention is unconscionable.

A user-friendly kiosk format should also be implemented to expedite the dissemination of information for application to the operational activities of the end-user. This information must be reliable, succinct, and intelligible. A process for gathering, analyzing, sharing, and managing incident-related information and intelligence must also be established. This intelligence information can come from a variety of sources, such as risk assessments, medical intelligence, weather information, utilities and public works data, geospatial data, structural designs, and toxic contaminant laboratory data.

In an information technology age that is rapidly evolving, it is critical to comprehend and utilize advanced information-based technologies. The interpretation of such information has increasingly dramatic impacts upon operational effectiveness and, ultimately, individual and community survival. There is also the potential to provide vital and essential information to law enforcement and security personnel as well as other responders for their interpretation and use distinct from the usual public health functions.

This information may also address, and empower, the users of public health information on intelligence, tactical, and operational levels in their efforts at maintaining national and domestic security and order. It can be used to inform and educate the general public on pressing public health matters, such as pandemics or food-borne illness outbreaks. Disaster and emergency response planning can be greatly enhanced through its use.

I am currently developing the public health fusion center concept. I will continue to expound upon this subject and its applications in future writings. What I have provided in this book is a description of various community-based elements and an explanation of new theories and elements within concepts I have developed. These points concern the composition and structure of the community settings. In the next chapter, I will discuss issues that arise when you find yourself within an event or incident that has arisen.

PART 5

In the Midst of Disaster

Chapter 16

The Incident or Event Which Goes Awry

Never before has the need for a formalized emergency response process been so greatly needed globally. The NIMS and ICS systems, described in *Chapter 13—NIMS and the Need for Preparedness*, laid the foundation for the requisite approach to meeting this need. The following discussion involves an overview of a response process that is heavily entrenched in the framework provided by the NIMS and ICS systems. At a bare minimum, the following is required during any operational intervention:

1. Clear-cut strategic goals
2. Deliverables and operating objectives
3. Definitive implementation strategies
4. Unequivocal specification of assignments and duty responsibilities
5. Measurable performance objectives

The concept of resiliency begins at the individual level. That is—you! Just as all disasters begin locally, so resiliency begins within the individual. Community members must respond collectively to the challenges of an incident, emergency, or event that goes awry. This response is predicated upon and orchestrated by individual responses within a community. A person's individual actions, or inactions, can worsen or improve the consequences arising from such response efforts – which are aimed at averting a poor outcome in any situation that threatens life or property.

COL. Damon T. Arnold, M.D., M.P.H.

Resiliency Begins at the Individual Level

The development of resiliency on a very fundamental level requires very little time. This time investment is priceless with respect to the sense of security, peace of mind, and confidence it confers upon the participant. What one is attempting to do in this process is to predict the possible challenges that will be faced within a disaster situation. Once this is ascertained, the individual must avoid or eliminate the destructive consequences arising from the situation at hand. Implementing such a policy consistently as it applies to routine life activities will lead to a more effective response during times of an emergency or disaster.

Proper nutrition and exercise as well as avoiding poor health-related behaviors not only can prevent the onset of injury, illness, and disease in one's lifetime but also increases one's chances for survival during an emergency or disaster. While I was involved in military operations, this was dramatically apparent to me. The U.S. Army makes a concerted effort to emphasize the need for physical fitness and proper discipline. When faced with adversity, those in excellent physical shape have a survival advantage over those who are not.

In addition, one should regularly make sure your personal and family members financial, insurance, and medical records are updated and prepared for potential use. This will save valuable time looking for and trying to gather information should an emergency or disaster situation arise. Making sure key family members know the location and have access to—and possibly already secured duplicate copies of—the documents is also important.

Establishing such a preparedness and resiliency posture on a community-wide basis requires this process to begin well before an emergency or disaster. Preparedness encompasses basic day-to-day survival skills and preparations one makes to avoid adverse outcomes within one's environment. It also includes one's degree of adaptability in meeting the needs of emergency and disaster situations. This stems from our very basic survival skills. Inaction at this basic level portends increased vulnerability and a failure to respond appropriately during a subsequent emergency or disaster situation. For instance, you should know in advance where to obtain information, alerts, advisories, and updates. You should also make sure you know how to interpret and understand what these communications mean. Also, have plans to respond to their directives. An all-encompassing perspective is required here.

Responding to an Emergency

If you are an emergency responder, managing resources safely and effectively is the most important consideration at a response site. Therefore, personnel and equipment should respond only when requested or when dispatched by an appropriate authority. Resources must be organized, assigned, and directed to accomplish the objectives. These elements must effectively respond to ever-changing conditions. Once again, I present a brief summary here of the principles covered in the FEMA course at www.fema.gov. You should complete this training if you have not already done so.

The creation and assembly of a mission-specific travel kit is a priority. You may wish to assemble a few of these kits, if possible, with one kept in your home, workplace, and car trunk. When a disaster or emergency occurs, you are statistically more likely to be at one of these sites. Since you can't be certain of your location when an emergency occurs, I recommend kits at all three of these sites if you feel it is feasible.

These kits should include personal care and sustenance items, mobile computing and communications devices, an emergency weather radio, a flashlight, a camping knife, a rope, an emergency whistle, hard copies of regional maps, contact lists, a blanket, emergency manuals, cash, and other essential equipment. A standard emergency kit for a car should always be maintained and can provide further resources during a response. You must guard these against theft and misuse. If you chose to place cash in the response kit, you must weigh this decision yourself. ATM machines may be depleted or non-functional during emergencies.

Remember that ATM machines may not be functioning during a disaster, and cash may be needed, as noted by General Russel Honore in his book entitled *Survival*.[5] This is a must read! He is not only a great general, but a rare prophetic voice on the subject of preparedness as well.

Ensure continued communication on a periodic basis with work associates and family members. This will help to minimize the stress of being away from your family and coworkers with whom you have formed relationships and mutual support. Make sure to review potential assignment roles and to check on travel authorizations and transportation arrangements as well as payroll status and procedures. This will minimize the need to respond to these issues in the middle of a response in which you may be heavily engaged.

Review your emergency role assignment and know who you will report to. Clearly understand what your position will be and the extent of your decision-making authority. Determine the correct communication procedures for contacting headquarters and other emergency response elements you will be interacting with.

You must also identify the purchasing authority and procedures for such transactions. Also identify procedures for obtaining food and lodging. I have witnessed situations where individuals arranged for lodging and food on their own. They then proceeded, only to find reimbursement was not authorized or allowed for those expenditures.

It is noted within the federal guidance on the NIMS that a deployment briefing should include at a minimum the following information:

1. Incident type and name or designation
2. Descriptive location and response area
3. Incident check-in location
4. Specific assignment
5. Reporting date and time
6. Travel instructions
7. Communications instructions

---

[5]   Lt. Geen. Russel Honore, *Survival* (Atria Books, 2009).

8. Special support required (facilities, equipment, transportation, off-loading, etc.)
9. Travel authorizations (air, rental car, lodging, meals, incidentals, etc.)

Upon arrival at the incident site, you are only to check-in once using the ICS Form 211, "Check-In List." This officially logs you in at the event and helps to accomplish the following objectives:

1. Ensure personal accountability.
2. Track resources.
3. Prepare personnel for assignments/reassignments.
4. Locate personnel in case of an emergency.
5. Establish time records and payroll documentation.
6. Plan for releasing personnel.
7. Organize the demobilization process.

Locate your incident supervisor and obtain your initial briefing, which should include the following:

1. Current situation assessment
2. Identification of your specific job responsibilities
3. Identification of coworkers
4. Location of work area
5. Identification of required eating and sleeping areas
6. Identify all needed accommodations for personal hygiene and bathroom needs
7. Procedural instructions for obtaining additional supplies, services and personnel
8. Operational periods/work shifts
9. Required safety procedures and PPE, as appropriate

All incidents require some form of recordkeeping. General guidelines for incident record keeping include the following:

1. Print or type all entries.
2. Enter dates in month/day/year format.
3. Use military 24-hour time.

4. Enter date and local time on all forms and records.
5. Fill in all the blanks, and use NA as appropriate.
6. Section chiefs and above assign a record keeper.

If you are expected to be a supervisor, you must maintain a daily Unit Log (ICS-214). This log must indicate the names of personnel assigned and a listing of the major activities that occurred during the operational periods to which you were assigned. You are expected to give briefings to your subordinates, adjacent forces, and replacement personnel.

Communication discipline is compulsory, and includes the following:

1. Observe strict radio/telephone procedures (official use *only!*).
2. Use plain English in all communications.
3. Codes should not be used for radio transmissions.
4. Limit radio and telephone traffic to essential information only, and plan what you will say before you attempt to speak.
5. Follow all communications security procedures.
6. Sexual harassment or discrimination of any type and the use of illegal drugs and/or alcohol are prohibited at all incident sites.
7. Be patient, act professionally, reduce stress, and pay attention to those adversely responding to stress.

General Demobilization Guidelines for all personnel, include the following:

1. Complete all work assignments and required forms and reports.
2. Brief supervisor, subordinates, and replacements.
3. Evaluate the performance of subordinates.
4. Follow incident and agency checkout procedures.
5. Provide adequate follow-up contact information.
6. Return any incident-issued equipment or other nonexpendable supplies.
7. Complete post-incident reports, critiques, evaluations, and medical follow-ups.
8. Complete all payment and/or payroll issues or obligations.

9. Contact the demobilization unit to obtain demobilization instructions and notify the home unit on return home.

ICS organizational structure deliberately differs from any already-existing agency administrative structure. This is intended to prevent confusion over reporting structures and various role assignments. There are five major management functional groupings:

1. Incident Command [only ICS position always staffed]
2. Finance/Administration Section
3. Logistics Section
4. Operations Section
5. Planning Section

I have found that these organizational and operational principles and concepts closely parallel those followed within military operational theatres. There should be a concerted effort to become familiar with the perspectives, skills, abilities, and talents that your team members bring to the table. This is where teamwork leads to cooperation, collaboration, and potential synergisms that make otherwise unobtainable goal accomplishments possible. You must also know your limitations and when to ask for assistance and report important findings to others as the situation evolves. Without effective communication, there is no unity of purpose or effort.

Your Personal Emergency Plan

This discussion describes some of the resources you should always have ready prior to an emergency or disaster response situation. It is a good idea to store at least two weeks of nonperishable foods. These items can be rotated and replaced with your regularly utilized nonperishable food items periodically. This is done to ensure that expiration dates are not exceeded during prolonged storage.

Food that is selected should not require refrigeration, preparation, or cooking. Likewise, foods having a high salt content or that require the addition of water should be avoided. Salty foods causing increased thirst and foods requiring water both can waste limited drinking water supplies. Include a manual can opener and reusable eating utensils. Also include formulas for infants and those with special nutritional needs. This includes those with medical illnesses, food allergies, and seniors. Include food for your pets as well.

It is also recommended that you store a two-week supply of water in the amount of one gallon per person per day. Half of this is to be used for drinking water and the other half for sanitary needs. Remember that children, seniors, nursing mothers, and those with illnesses generally need more water for their daily needs. Of course, pets also require water. Fluids with electrolytes are a benefit in situations where high temperatures prevail, as sweating can deplete your body of required electrolytes. When I was deployed in Iraq, it became apparent that in regions where there are extremely high temperatures, individuals may not appear to be sweating at all. This is because of the rapid evaporation of sweat. They are still losing large amounts of fluid, even though the sweat is not visible. The person is becoming dehydrated and overheated and is potentially becoming severely dehydrated. Therefore, the absence of sweat is a very worrisome sign in extremely hot conditions.

Avoid using glass bottles that may break and easily degradable containers. I keep a water filter and iodine tablets in my personal emergency kits. You should be aware of water boiling instructions. Protect your food and water sources from contamination by environmental agents and wild animals.

In disaster environments, remember that wild animals may intrude into areas where they do not normally tread. Once the environment is disrupted, the human boundaries of city and rural environments may be degraded or no longer exist. This allows for the transmigration of animals and organisms into human environments. Therefore, dispose of all leftover foods and trash appropriately. Do not leave it lying around, as it will attract animals. The general rule is that rats follow trash, and snakes follow rats. I can guarantee you that you do not want to be a part of this picture.

Sanitation is of the utmost importance in such an environment. Garbage bags, tissues, toilet paper, and wet wipes are a great help and should be handled and disposed of properly. Wet wipes should be fragrance free, so as to avoid attracting biting insects. Disposable diapers should be included for infants. Soap and alcohol-based hand-washing solutions are very useful and should be included in your kits. Avoid direct sunlight in open areas if it is hot. Keep sunglasses and a lightweight hat in the emergency kit. I also keep safety goggles in my kits in case I have to traverse wooded areas with tree branches or windy terrains with blowing debris. Eye protection is essential in these environments.

Make sure to also include a portable radio that runs on batteries, electricity, solar power, and which has a hand-crank for recharging. There are several available for use, including the American Red Cross models, which I currently have on hand and which are excellent. Also, keep a flashlight that utilizes several power types to operate. Solar-powered and cranked devices are preferable. Batteries and electrical power may not be available during a situation where social disruption is rampant.

It is essential that you prepare emergency supply kits that include needed equipment and supplies for health and medical needs. You should stock at least one month of all required prescription medications and emergency medical supplies for yourself and family members as well. This includes over-the-counter anti-allergy medications, antacids, anti-diarrhea medications, a non-breakable thermometer, and medications for fever and/or pain. Make sure to check for contraindications to taking medications, such as medicinal allergies or medical conditions. Be sure to keep up with replacing expired medications in the emergency kit.

Sunscreen is a must for anyone in a hot environment. Also, include a blanket, as this may be required in cool or cold weather. Remember to safeguard all medical supplies and medications, especially with children. Again, keep copies of all health records for easy access throughout any emergency or disaster. It is important to address all your usual medical needs and also those that could arise during a disaster. There are many lists of suggested disaster supplies. I recommend that you review several of these documents. It is also important to determine what works for you and what you have learned from prior educational, exercise, drill, or real-life experiences.

Entering the arena of response and recovery operations requires preparation on the part of the participant if that person is to provide a significant contribution to the process. I always keep a daily activity log of issues and findings when on missions. Often these writings have been entered into after-action reports and have aided me in refining my approaches to subsequent mission assignments.

In the next chapter, I describe the process of recovery, which still is difficult to fully define or comprehend. It is also a concept in need of a great deal of further attention.

Chapter 17

Recovery—Beyond the Midst of Disaster

Social disruption recovery processes revolve around two perspectives, noted in earlier chapters. First is an automatic tendency to want to describe recovery as beginning and arising within the context of a man-made or natural disaster aftermath. However, recovery begins with the steps made toward ensuring social and CIKR stability, resiliency, and preparedness in the pre-disaster or pre-emergency situation. Secondly, if the strengthening of community infrastructure, resilience capabilities, and the state of readiness at all times is not ensured, one enters an uphill battle in both the response and recovery efforts.

You would never think of entering an athletic event or musical instrument performance competition without preparation, training, and practice. Surely, you would be clobbered on the field by a more experience athlete and upstaged by a well-rehearsed and trained musical virtuoso. So why should you expect to enter the response or recovery phase after an emergency, disaster, or poor event outcome and expect to excel in response and recovery without proper preparation, training, and practice drills?

As noted earlier, there is always a certain level of social disruption or disorder present within a community at any given point in time. Also, there are more vulnerable subpopulations within these settings. These various levels of disorder should be assessed and addressed to eliminate such disparities, preferably before the need for a disaster response arises. During a disaster response, attention should be paid to the entire community's population base. This is in order to stabilize the community base and to make it more resilient to the disruptive forces that have arisen or will continue to arise. Prepare for a community-based emergency, disaster, or poor event outcome by ensuring that you have taken steps to react appropriately to these situations. This will bring confidence and a certain level of calmness to such situations and those around you. You will be more effective in addressing issues that tend to arise.

It is essential that you know in advance where to get information about advisories, emergency plans, updates, and alerts. You must also understand what this information means and how to use it in your response role. This also sets the stage for recovery efforts. During a prolonged recovery period, the preparation of needed supplies can have tremendous impacts on your potential for survival.

During the recovery period, safety is the first and most important step. For example, if you are not qualified to do so, do not attempt to repair electrical lines in standing water. This may seem ridiculous, and it is. However, people have attempted things like this before in disaster situations with terrible results. There are many situations, such as the use of various power tools that are dangerous in unskilled hands, which can result in a worsening of the situation or downright tragedies. Do not add to the burdens placed upon your response team by becoming a victim yourself. Know your limitations and skill sets. Note that the effectiveness of your skills and abilities may be altered or negatively impacted by the disrupted and unfamiliar situation you find yourself within.

The emotional and spiritual dimensions that arise in these settings are also tremendously important to address properly. Counseling and spiritual guidance can have an incredible impact on the recovery process for those who have been traumatized by the unfolding catastrophe they are experiencing. These destructive acts not only affect a person's present circumstances, but work to destroy their past memories, hopes, dreams, and plans. It is essential that victims of such disasters become actively involved in the recovery process and that the resources they need to make a recovery are provided to them. Realize the impact of these circumstances on your team members as well. Since all disasters begin locally, the team members are likely to be acting in a community of which they are an integral part. This makes them more likely to be affected by the psychosocial consequences of such a disrupted environment. This is especially true if they intimately know the people affected.

Recovery Is a Puzzle of Varied and Complex Views

We are living during a time when it seems as if each unfolding day presents us with another disaster situation. To address the issue of recovery, we first must sketch the scene of what things were like in a community prior to the disaster. This can be difficult for you to accomplish, especially if you are in an unfamiliar environment. It may also be difficult for those who live within the disaster zone to put into words what has happened and what was there before. Recovery is a puzzle of varied and complex views of what reality was like prior to the occurrence of the disaster—that is, how that reality is viewed by inhabitants within the affected community.

The goal of recovery must be tied to these views despite the difficulties they present for the responders. The prioritization of recovery objectives, and the steps to be taken, can be deeply affected by the views and wishes of the community members involved in the process. Their wishes must be respected. Guidance concerning operational issues must be fully explained to these community members. This is extremely important to do when a deviation from their view is contemplated and envisioned by the response team.

During Katrina, I and the team went to the aid a gentleman and his wife at their badly stricken home. His request was for me and the accompanying soldiers to help him move his boat out of his backyard. At first, this seemed like a strange request. His wife looked me straight in the eyes and said, "Please, just do it for him." Once we accomplished the task, he breathed a great sigh of relief, feeling he had begun to reestablish order in his life.

The gentleman's wife was spot-on; she realized that this act would allow her husband to deal with the unfolding disaster. It is important to keep in mind that you are helping survivors to reestablish their sense of order, not yours. The steps they feel they need to take may be critical in their personal recovery process. One must also keep in mind that not all requests can be met as resource shortfalls, imminent danger, or more pressing priorities may emerge.

The issue of recovery received little if any attention in the past. This may be due to the protracted nature of recovery and the great need for additional fiscal and other resources that must be met for it to be fully actualized. Despite this, recovery has begun to gain more attention recently. Many of the sites of tragic disasters over the past two decades are still far from being fully recovered. The restoration of critical infrastructure and key resource sectors in these communities have been challenging at best.

In addition, some of these sites move from one disaster scenario to the next, with little intervening time for true recovery to occur. It is especially important for such areas to become increasingly resilient as they rebuild their environments so as to mitigate the impact of any future disasters. The essential elements for community rebuilding with resiliency in mind provides fertile ground for creative and innovative solutions. This was accomplished with modifications in the construction of buildings in California earthquake zones. The buildings were made more resistant to earthquakes.

It should be required that a detailed analysis of every community be made prior to potential disasters. The more complete this picture is with respect to a reflection of the predisaster status of a community, the better it will serve the purpose for setting a recovery endpoint. This requires the reestablishment of normal or near-normal infrastructure support mechanisms and operations. It also calls for the implementation of a sustainable mechanism to complete an acceptable outcome.

Such an undertaking truly requires community-wide effort and relies upon a broad-based collaborative environment. Care must be taken not to overshadow the community members' ultimate wishes in the recovery process. Recovery must receive more attention as an integral part of overall response efforts.

Throughout the history of this country, it has been exactly during such times that the American spirit and ingenuity have shined through. During our darkest moments in history, we have found solutions for our deepest and most complex societal problems. Today is no different. Resolve and dedication to service should serve as the launching pad for positive movements in a health-conscious direction for our collective society and nation.

Epilogue

I created the Theory of Social Disruption model to form a perspective on the societal dynamics that are operating on a community-based level during times of quiescence as well as disaster. It illustrates the fact that often the borderlines between what does and does not constitute a disaster or emergency are artificially and poorly drawn. The model also offers a functional framework upon which one can place and measure operational intervention strategies—during both routine and disaster response efforts. The suggested use of the medical home kiosk model is just one potential application of an intervention strategy, as is the public health fusion center model. Both of these concepts are based upon an understanding of the Theory of Social Disruption modeling I presented. I will be exploring the use of these tools in future writings.

Further, this Theory of Social Disruption lends itself to the inclusion and application of mathematical analyses. Such an approach can involve the use of performance metrics and health impact assessments to determine the effectiveness of various implementation strategies. This will allow the capture of invaluable data during routine public health operations as well as during response efforts aimed at evolving, scalable social disruptions. The mathematical analyses can include the application of the principles of epidemiology, accounting, and higher mathematics. The purpose for this is the measurement, further delineation, and refinement of rational, community-based implementation strategies. These strategies should be directed at the elimination of disparities and the strengthening of general community stability and resiliency.

The mantra and battle cry of the current fiscal age is 'no metrics, no money.' Unfortunately, many positive intervention benefits can become obscured by a system bent purely upon immediate fiscal outcomes. This is because such a policy position pays little attention to the total impact a disruptive occurrence involving an individual community member can have on society as a whole. For example, what would happen if a policy decision was made not to fund emergency response elements that normally cover car accidents? If a three-car accident completely shut down a major highway entering a city, a tendency to focus on only the cars involved exists. If emergency response services were unavailable, the untrained occupants of nearby cars may attempt to respond, putting themselves in danger. However, the delay creates a backed-up traffic flow pattern that may last hours, due to the lack of trained professionals at the accident scene. This prevents the material resources and professionals—such as raw materials, bankers, doctors, and laborers required for normal business operations—from reaching the city's interior.

Such a situation will result in millions, if not billions, of dollars in economic damage—which is astronomical compared to the price of having a response crew readily available to rectify the accident situation. As a result, this policy would put the economy of the community at greater risk of financial loss and harm due to the implementation of poor fiscal policy practices.

This underscores the fact that the funding for emergency response activities should never be compromised. However, shortsighted policies such as the one noted would compromise our national and domestic security.

Such a policy approach also misses the human dimensions of emotional, mental, and spiritual well-being, and cultural significance. These dimensions form the very basis and the reason why society exists in the first place. The existence of society is generally based upon mutual, interpersonal support that imparts a greater degree of social stability and survivability for its collective members.

Our policies should support the Constitutional perspective of a fundamental equality of all people within our country. These policies need to apply resources equitably and consistent with the relative needs of those afflicted. This should be done with respect to all who are at any risk of pain, suffering, or premature mortality. Moral and ethical principles that reflect the best intentions and results for all members of this nation should be applied. To avoid the issue of disparities and to do less is frankly immoral, unethical, and fundamentally unconstitutional. This was a challenge presented to American citizens by the signatories of the American Constitution.

Further, the medical community and society as a whole have done an abysmal job at addressing the emotional, mental, and spiritual dimensions of the needs of community members. I was giving a keynote speech recently and asked a question to over 300 hundred in attendance. They all had impressive academic credentials and professional degrees. I asked to see the hand of anyone in the room who had ever had a course in how to be a happy, successful, and healthy person in our society. Not one hand arose in response. This is a sad comment on how we operate as a society with respect to our educational experiences and policy directives. It also demonstrates the disregard for the value placed upon and the investments made in the health and happiness of our citizens.

Unfortunately, this orientation repeatedly appears during the application of social policies. There is often a disregard for the destructive side effects imposed by ill-conceived intervention strategies or harmful legislative policy decisions. Not only do they fail to address the person as a whole, they very often create an imposed sense of helplessness and lack of self-sufficiency on the part of the recipients. This worsens the situation for community members. At best this is an unconstitutional, immoral, and unethical practice.

Future perspectives on this dynamic process as well as innovation will be required to create the most effective approaches to solve the problems of community-based instability. However, as I stated before, one must never stray too far from anything less than a strong degree of community engagement. It is essential to gain community input for solutions to societal problems. Why are we living in this society if not for a healthy and happy life as well as mutual support?

When I was in office as a state public health director for only two weeks, a legislator asked me how it felt to be on the top of the public health pyramid. I replied by explaining that the pyramid must be turned upside down, as the strongest part of the pyramid is the base—that is, the people that support our society. The top of the pyramid is there only because the people decided to have one. A public servant must always remember that the people are what matters most and act accordingly, with both morals and ethics. The preamble to the United States Constitution begins with the powerful words 'We the People.' This thought should be kept in mind when formulating any public health intervention strategy. It is the people that we work for.

Glossary of Terms

Accessible: The presence of the requisite and legally mandated features and qualities that ensure easy infrastructure entrance and utilization, which allows participation and use of programs, services, activities, and facilities by individuals with a wide variety of disabilities.

Acquisition procedures: A process by which one obtains the requisite resources for supporting operational resource requirements.

Agency dispatch: The agency or selected jurisdictional facility from which resources are distributed to incident sites.

All-hazards approach: An incident or emergency, natural or man-made, which warrants action to protect life, property, the environment, and public health or safety, and to minimize disruptions of government, social, or economic activities.

Area command: An organizational structure established to manage multiple incidents that are being handled by separate Incident Command Systems or multiple incident management teams. The establishment of an area command is contingent upon need, span of control, and incident complexity considerations.

Assessment: Monitoring, collecting, processing, analyzing, evaluating, and interpreting data and intelligence information. It attempts to put into a real-time perspective the various observations and information obtained in order to guide the decision-making process and operational intervention strategies contemplated.

Assignment: The task(s) provided to specified resource personnel, for them to perform within an operational period. The task is based upon the Incident Action Plan's stated operational objectives.

Assistant: The title for subordinates of principal command staff member positions who may also be assigned to unit leaders. The assistant provides direct support, advice, and subject matter expertise to his or her superiors and has qualifications and technical capabilities commensurate with his or her level of subordinate responsibility.

Assisting agency: Any agency that directly provides personnel, services, or other resources to another agency that is charged with direct authority and responsibility for incident management of an incident situation.

Available resource: A resource that has been assigned to an incident and checked in as available for a mission assignment. The available resource is usually maintained in the staging area.

Badging: This is the process of assigning incident-specific credentials to establish the legitimacy of responding participants which serves to provide or limit access to various specific incident site locations.

Base: A base is where primary logistics and administrative functions are coordinated and administered (only one base is allowed per incident).

Branch: The organizational level charged with functional or geographic responsibility for major aspects of incident operations. Branches are denoted by their functional area or by roman numerals.

Cache: A predetermined complement of required tools, equipment, and supplies stored in a designated storage location that is available for incident use.

Camp: A geographical site within the general incident area (separate from the incident base) that is equipped and staffed to provide food, water, sanitary services, and sleeping accommodations to incident personnel. The campsite is designated by geographic location or by a number.

Certifying personnel: This is the process of authoritatively attesting to the fact that individual responders meet the professional, educational, training, and experience requirements and standards for their stated position.

Chain of command: An orderly line of authority within the ranks of the incident management organization.

Check-in process: The report-in process where one registers one's presence and receives an assignment. This is required for all responders, regardless of their affiliations or role, and each individual must receive an assignment in accordance with the procedures established by the Incident commander.

Chief: The Incident Command System (ICS) title bestowed upon an individual who is responsible for the management of a functional section. These functional sections include operations, planning, logistics, finance/administration, and, if it is established as a separate section, intelligence/investigations.

Common Integrated Communications Plan: This includes equipment, protocols, procedures, and systems that operate across jurisdictions prior to an incident or event. Effective ICS communications include three elements: modes, planning, and networks (internal and external).

Command: The empowerment of an individual to act via directing, ordering, or controlling by virtue of explicit statutory, regulatory, or delegated authority.

Command staff: Staff members who report directly to the incident commander. It includes the safety officer, public information officer, liaison officer, and other positions as deemed necessary by the incident commander. Each of these staff members may also have assigned assistants as well.

Common operating picture: An overview of an incident by all relevant parties that provides incident information enabling the incident commander or unified command and any supporting agencies and organizations to make effective, consistent, and timely decisions.

Common terminology: The use of commonly recognized terms across multiple areas of discipline so as to avoid misunderstandings, misinterpretations, and confusion.

Communications: The sharing of information through verbal, written, visual, tactile, or symbolic modes of information transfer presentation.

Communications/dispatch center: Information and resource dispatch centers, 911 emergency call centers, and established emergency command-and-control centers. This can serve the purpose of a centralized, primary coordination and support element of the Multiagency Coordination Systems (MACS) until other elements of the MACS are formally established.

Complex: A situation in which there are two or more individual incidents in the same general area and are assigned to a single incident commander or unified command.

Continuity of Operations Plan (COOP): The COOP involves the creation of a response plan within individual organizations that ensures the primary mission's essential functions continue be performed despite the occurrence of an incident or emergency situation.

Cooperating agency: This provides assistance other than direct operational or support functions or resources to the incident management effort.

Coordinate: To assist in the balancing of priorities and demands placed upon response elements within the operating environment. This also involves advancing the systematic sharing of information, analyses, and a common operational vision among principals who know or have a need to know, in order to carry out their specific incident management responsibilities.

Corrective actions: The implementation of procedures that are based on lessons learned from actual incidents or from training and exercises. These commonly arise in After Action Reviews (AARs).

Credentialing: This is the process of verifying and authenticating the identity and certification status of designated incident site managers and emergency responders.

Critical infrastructure: Recognized concrete or virtual assets, systems, and networks that are so vital to societal stability that their incapacitation or destruction would exert a debilitating effect upon local or even national safety, security, economic stability, or public health outcomes.

Delegation of authority: A statement to the incident commander by the agency executive delegating authority and assigning responsibility. This delegation of authority can also delineate expectations, objectives, priority concerns, constraints, or other points of guidance deemed necessary by the delegating authority. Agencies often require this to be formalized in a Letter of Expectation to officially authenticate this delegation of authority prior to the incident commander assuming his or her role as commander.

Demobilization: The orderly, efficient, and safe return of an incident resource to its location of origin.

Department Operations Center (DOC): An Emergency Operations Center (EOC) specific to a single department or agency. The focus of a DOC is upon an internal department or agency-specific incident management and response. It is often linked to and represented within a combined multiagency EOC by authorized agents for the originating department or agency.

Deputy: A fully qualified individual who, in the absence of a superior for whatever reason, can be delegated the authority required to manage or perform a specific function or task. Such deputies generally can be assigned to the incident commander, general staff, and branch directors.

Director: The Incident Command System title applies to branch supervisors.

Dispatching: This is the orderly communication and movement of a resource or resources to an assigned operational mission location. This may also involve an administrative movement from one location to another.

Division: The organizational level having responsibility for operations within a defined geographic area. These are often established when the number of resources existing within an environment exceeds the available manageable span of control of the section chief.

Emergency: Any incident or derailed event that requires responsive action to protect life, limb, or property. Within the purview of the Robert T. Stafford Disaster Relief and Emergency Assistance Act, an emergency means any occasion or instance for which, in the determination of the United States, federal assistance is needed to supplement state and local efforts and capabilities to save lives and to protect property and public health and safety, or to lessen or avert the threat of a catastrophe in any part of the United States.

Emergency Management Assistance Compact (EMAC): A congressionally ratified organization that provides form and structure to interstate mutual aid. Through EMAC, a disaster-impacted state may request and receive assistance from other member states quickly and efficiently. In the process, the key issues of reimbursement and liability are addressed and resolved.

Emergency Operations Center (EOC): The temporary or permanent physical location where response personnel coordinate the resources and information flows in support of on-scene operational activities. It may be organized around a specific federal, state, or local jurisdiction or a response element theme such as fire control, medical service provision, or concerns for ensuring security.

Emergency Operations Plan (EOP): An ongoing plan responding to a wide variety of potential hazardous situations.

Emergency Support Function (ESF): A series of various groupings of private-sector and governmental capabilities into supportive organizational structures that provide resources and services to meet the needs arising at the incident response sites. ESF-8 specifically addresses the health and medical services that are provided during a response effort that is directed through the assistant secretary for health, who serves as the executive agent for the Department of Health and Human Services (DHHS).

Emergency public information: Emergency public information includes information just prior to, during, or in the aftermath of a disaster that provides directives for taking action or situational awareness.

Evacuation: The phased, organized, and supervised withdrawal, dispersal, or removal of civilians from dangerous or potentially dangerous locations to safer areas where they can be received and acquire care.

Event: A planned, scheduled, nonemergency occurrence or activity such as a sporting event, family outing, concert, cultural fair, or parade.

Federal: Anything of or pertaining to the federal government of the United States of America and its territories.

Field Operations Guide: A durable pocket or desk guide that contains essential written information and often visual aids to assist in the performance of specific tasks, functions, and assigned duties.

Finance/administration section: The Incident Command System section responsible for all administrative and financial considerations surrounding an incident.

Function: The five major activities in the Incident Command System: command, operations, planning, logistics, and finance/administration.

General staff: Usually consists of planning, operations, logistics, and finance/administration section chiefs and reports to the incident commander. It may also include an intelligence/investigations section chief if desired by the incident commander.

Group: An organization subdivision initiated in order to divide the incident management structure into functional areas of operation. These groups are comprised of resources that are aligned to perform a special function not necessarily within a single geographic division.

Hazard: An agent or circumstance that is potentially harmful or dangerous and often serves as the root cause of a negative outcome.

Heli-base (fueling and routine maintenance) and heli-spot (temporary): The areas from which a helicopter's operations are conducted.

Hospital Incident Command System (HICS): HICS, which is an ICS-based system, is the standard for hospital-based incident management. Hospital implementation of HICS ensures compliance with NIMS objectives 7, 11, and 12. The hospital still has to comply with other NIMS principles regarding communications, resources management, training and exercises, and preparedness not covered under the HICS.

Incident: A natural or man-made occurrence that results in the need for a response in order to save life, limb, or property. This includes, for example, transportation accidents, natural weather and geological disturbances, wartime and terrorist activities, famine, and public health emergencies.

Incident Command: Composed of the incident commander and assigned supporting staff members and is charged with the management of the incident response efforts.

Incident Command Post (ICP): Provides for easy access and communication at a site close to the incident site and contains a meeting area located outside of existing physical hazard areas.

Incident Command System (ICS): An on-scene, standardized, and integrated organizational management system that forms in response to single or multiple scalable incidents of varying degrees of complexity without regard to jurisdictional boundaries. ICS aligns and manages personnel, facilities, equipment, procedures, and equipment within a common organizational response structure. This approach is widely used in both public and private sector settings.

Incident commander (IC): This individual has authority and responsibility for all response activities, including management and operations at the incident site. The IC is responsible for the development of strategies and tactics as well as the ordering and release of resources.

Incident management: Involves the full spectrum of public-private partnerships that collaborate to provide for planned, integrated, efficient, coordinated, and supportive response and recovery effort outcomes. This is regardless of the ultimate cause, size, or complexity of the incident(s).

Incident management team (IMT): Comprised of the incident commander and the appropriate command and general staff personnel assigned to an incident. The 'type' or 'level' of IMT formed depends on the qualifications, training, and experience of the IMT personnel and the identified formal response responsibilities and needs that are addressed.

Incident objectives: Incident objectives are explicit directives and guidance provided to personnel that is required to select appropriate strategies and direct tactical resource utilizations. The incident objectives must be realistic, achievable, and measurable. They must also be flexible enough to adapt to incident-related situational changes that require alternative strategies and tactical responses.

Information management: Information management involves the collection, organization, analysis, and validation of information and intelligence. Consistency in messaging must be established. The information and intelligence must be processed and prepared for distribution to the appropriate stakeholder venues.

Integrated Planning System: The integrated planning system was designed to provide a unified and comprehensive process approach to the development and integration of plans for federal government agencies. This is consistent with the expectations noted in the Homeland Security Management System as outlined in the National Strategy for Homeland Security.

Intelligence/investigations: This information leads to the detection and prevention of a criminal or terrorist act or provides for the identification, apprehension, interrogation, and prosecution of suspected or known criminals and terrorists.

Interoperability: This involves the ability of two or more systems to provide, receive, and exchange communications, data, resources, and equipment in order for them to operate effectively together. Such interoperability can exist within the public, private, or public-private partnership domains.

Job aid: Includes checklists, visual cues, signs, or symbols that are aimed at ensuring the accomplishment of tasks or assignments.

Joint Field Office (JFO): The primary location of the federal incident management field structure. This is a temporary office for the central coordination of federal, state, local, tribal, territorial, private sector, and nongovernmental responder organizations. It operates according to NIMS principles, and a JFO is present to provide support, not to manage, response element activities.

Joint Information Center (JIC): Established to coordinate all incident-related public information activities, it serves as the central point of contact for all news media and participating public information officers.

Joint Information System (JIS): Integrates collected incident-related information and public affairs activities into a cohesive organizational structure. The JIS strives to provide consistent, coordinated, accurate, accessible, timely, and complete information during the time of an emerging crisis or incident operations. It also creates recommended media strategies for the IC and aims at controlling rumors or inaccurate information that could undermine operational efficiency and erode public trust in the response efforts.

Jurisdiction: A range or sphere of authority over an area of concern, which can be in terms of political or geographical boundary lines as well as functional areas of expertise, such as public health.

Jurisdictional agency: An agency which has jurisdiction and responsibility for a specific geographical area or mandated function.

Key resource: Any privately or publicly controlled resource that has been deemed to be essential to the minimal operations of the government or the economy.

Letter of Expectation: This is a letter from the agency executive to the incident commander that delegates them authority and assigns them responsibility for all incident response efforts.

Liaison: A form of communication that strives to establish and maintain mutual understanding and cooperation while dealing with barriers to effective communication.

Liaison officer: A command staff member who is responsible for coordinating with representatives from cooperating and assisting agencies and organizations.

Local government: Public entities that are responsible for both the security and welfare of a designated area as established by law.

Logistics: The process and procedure for the provision of resources and services in support of incident management.

Logistics section: The incident command section charged with providing facilities, services, and materiel support for the incident.

Management by Objectives: A five-step management process approach for achieving an incident goal. This process includes establishing overarching incident objectives; developing strategies based upon these overarching incident objectives; developing and issuing assignments, plans, procedures, and protocols; establishing specific, measurable tactics or tasks for various incident-management strategic functional activities and directing efforts for their accomplishment; and collecting data and reports to measure and document performance and to facilitate the creation and implementation of corrective action steps.

Manager: An individual who is assigned specific managerial responsibilities within an ICS organizational unit.

Mitigation: The act of mitigation attempts to reduce or eliminate the loss of life, further injuries, and property damage that result from the occurrence of a man-made or natural disaster. It may be focused on efforts for developing resiliency or at breaking the cycle of disaster damage followed by reconstruction and then by repeated damage as occurs with repeated hurricanes or floods.

Mobilization: The process or procedures utilized by any organization for the activation, assembly, and transporting of requested and required resources in response to or in support of the occurrence of an incident.

Mobilization Guide: An outline of procedures, processes, and agreements utilized by all participating response agencies and organizations in achieving the activation, assembly, and transporting of resources.

Multi-Agency Coordination (MAC) group: This is a group with the authority or delegated authority to commit agency or organizational resources and funds. The MAC group can coordinate the decision making, use priority setting, and harmonize agency policy for the participating agencies. It can also provide guidance and direction in support of incident management activities. MAC groups may also be termed multiagency or emergency management committees.

Multi-Agency Coordination System (MACS): MACS provide assistance to organizations and agencies involved in incident response activities. A multi-agency coordination system serves as a platform for the coordination of incident-related priorities, communications, and information systems integration, and for making decisions concerning critical resource allocations. MACS include the elements of facilities, equipment, personnel, procedures, and communications within their organizational architecture.

Multijurisdictional incident: Response efforts often require an approach with components that arise within multiple jurisdictions to adequately respond to incident-related response issues and needs. The ICS dictates that these incidents be managed under a unified command structure that coordinates the contributions made by various jurisdictions to the overall response efforts.

Mutual aid agreement or assistance agreement: An oral or written mutual agreement between agencies, organizations, private partners, or jurisdictions that establishes a mechanism for the rapid and orderly acquisition and procurement of assistance in emergency and disaster response and recovery situations. This may include facilities, equipment, personnel, the provision of services, or any other required materiel need.

National: All levels of governance, policy, and existing infrastructure and resource sectors throughout the nation.

National Academies: Serve as advisers to the nation on the topics of science, engineering, and medicine. It is comprised of the National Academy of Science, the National Academy of Engineering, the Institute of Medicine, and the National Research Council.

National essential functions: A grouping of governmental functions related to the sustainment of national leadership and government institutional operability as the nation faces periods of disaster or catastrophic emergency.

National Incident Management System (NIMS): Homeland Security Presidential Directive-5 (HSPD-5), issued on November 28, 2003, set the stage for the creation of a consistent nationwide and proactive approach to address man-made and natural emergencies, disasters, and incidents. This provided the basis for federal, state, local and tribal governments, private sector entities, and nongovernmental organizations to work together to prepare for, respond to, and mitigate the harmful effects of and recover from domestic emergencies, disasters, and incidents that threaten life, property, or the environment—regardless of their origin, cause, size, or innate degree of complexity. NIMS contains core concepts, principles, and standardized, plain language terminology.

National Response Framework (NRF): The guiding principles that enable all response partners to prepare for and provide a unified, all-hazards national response effort to disasters and emergencies that are of national significance. It defines the roles, principles, and structures that organize the overall national response efforts. This builds upon the NIMS and provides for coordination and authorities within the context of a national response effort. The NRF replaced the National Response Plan (NRP) on March 22, 2008.

Nongovernmental organization (NGO): An organizational structure based upon the common interests of its members, which reside in the public sector. Although they may work with governmental entities, they are not a part of the government structure. They do not work to directly support a private interest. This includes the American Red Cross, faith-based institutions, and volunteer organizations. They often offer physical or psychological support services during emergency and disaster situations.

Officer: An ICS title given to the personnel responsible for one of the command staff positions of safety, liaison, or public information.

Operational period: An established time period, usually 12 or 24 hours, for the execution and accomplishment of a set of operational actions specified in the Incident Action Plan (IAP).

Operations section: The ICS section responsible for IAP implementation and all tactical operations.

Organization: Any association or group of individuals that organizes around a common interest or objective.

Personal responsibility: A responder's duty and obligation to be accountable for his or her actions.

Personnel accountability: The ability to determine the location and wellness status of incident personnel. Supervisors must ensure that ICS principles, processes, and guidelines as well as all response efforts are established and functioning properly.

Plain language: The use of plain language implies communications that can be understood by the intended audience, meet the purpose of information exchange, and leave little if any room for misinterpretation. Consistent with NIMS principles, it attempts to eliminate the use of code words, acronyms, and slang during incident responses. This is especially important when more than one agency or discipline is involved.

Planning meeting: A meeting convened whenever required and at any point within the response period. The meeting allows for the selection of appropriate strategies and tactics for incident control operations and for support and services efforts planning.

Planning section: Incident Command System planning section members shoulder the primary responsibility for the collection and evaluation of disaster and incident-related information. This is in order to amass the requisite information and intelligence for formulating a plan. They are also responsible for the ultimate construction and dissemination of the Incident Action Plan (IAP). This section is also responsible for maintaining information on situational awareness, forecasting, and assigned resource status updates.

Portability: An approach that facilitates the transferability of one or more components from one system to another distinctly different system while maintaining the components' operability and functionality—for example, transferring a program application from a laptop computer to a cell phone.

Prepositioned resource: The movement and placement of one or more given resource close to an area of anticipated or expected use.

Preparedness: A continuous, coordinated, and never-ending cycle of planning, procedures and protocol development, training, exercising, drilling, resources qualifications and certifications compliance checks, and evaluations with the purpose of taking necessary corrective steps. The process must be consistent with NIMS and ICS principles. The aim is to be prepared to respond at all times to an emergent disaster, emergency, or incident.

Prevention: Efforts at prevention are directed at preventing an incident from occurring or worsening and rely on such countermeasures and deterrence focuses activities as enhanced surveillance, inspections, security measures, public health interventions, and law enforcement and policing activities. The aim is to deter, preempt, interdict, disrupt, or eliminate illegal activity and apprehend potential criminals or terrorists and bring them to justice.

Predesignated incident locations: It is important to know the names and functions of principle predesignated incident locations. These are identified and established by the incident commander. The requirements vary depending on the resource needs and complexity of the incident or event.

Private sector: Formal or informal businesses, organizations, or individuals that are distinct from any governmental structure and includes for-profit and nonprofit organizations, commerce-related entities, and industries of various types.

Project Bio-shield Act: This act was signed by President Bush on July 21, 2004. It was enacted to accelerate the research, development, purchase, and availability of effective medical countermeasures against biological, chemical, radiological, and nuclear agents.

Protocol: A set of established guidelines for the implementation of specific interventions under specified conditions or circumstances. They may be applicable at an individual or a specified organizational level.

Public Health Emergency Medical Countermeasures Enterprises (PHEMCE): A coordinated effort through the Office of the Assistant Secretary for Preparedness and Response (ASPR), which coordinated an interagency initiative among the centers for Disease Control and Prevention (CDC), Food and Drug Administration (FDA), and the National Institutes of Health (NIH). With respect to the medical countermeasures, the PHEMCE:

- Defines and prioritizes requirements
- Integrates and coordinates research, product development, and procurement activities
- Sets deployment and uses strategies for the Strategic National Stockpile (SNS)
- Addresses CBRNE and naturally emerging infectious diseases and pandemic threats

Public information officer: This is a member of the command staff responsible for interacting with agencies, the public, and a multitude of media sources to determine information requirements and to communicate incident-related information.

Recovery: The development, coordination, and implementation of restoration plans for medical care access, CIKR sectors, economic stability, and resiliency for possible future disasters or incidents.

Resource management: Processes for categorizing, ordering, dispatching, tracking, and recovering resources. The resource management process allows the ordering and dispatch process, which spans across all levels of operation in both governmental, public, and private sectors, and ensures the appropriateness of resource utilization.

Resources: Includes personnel, supplies, equipment, and facilities that are, or are potentially, available for use during response and recovery efforts. Resources are described by type and kind.

Response: This involves the activities that address the short-term, direct effects of an incident or disaster. A response is focused upon saving life, limb, property, and the environment while attempting to meet the basic human needs of all those involved.

Safety officer: A member of the command staff who is charged with monitoring the incident operations and advising the incident commander on all matters relating to operational safety for responders and those within the operational area.

Single command: The incident commander has the complete and single command responsibility for incident management via the use of a single resource or a complex incident management team.

Situation report: Contains confirmed or verified information or intelligence regarding specific incident-related details.

Span of control: A key to effective and efficient incident management. This pertains to the number of individuals or other resources that one supervisor can manage effectively during emergency response incidents or special events. Safety and accountability are a top priority. The type of incident, nature of the task, hazards and safety factors, and distances between personnel and resources all influence span of control considerations. Effective span of control during incidents may vary from a maximum of three to seven elements reporting to a single supervisor, with five reporting elements being recommended as optimum.

Special needs population: A subpopulation of individuals who may have special needs based on, for example, poverty, disability status, age, language barriers, transportation needs, or special medical or care supervision requirements.

Staging area: A temporary holding area for resources prior to their tactical, operational assignment.

Standard Operating Guidelines (SOG): A set of instructions that have the force of a directive and cover those features of operations lending themselves toward definite or standardized procedures without loss of operational effectiveness.

Standardized Operating Procedure (SOP): This includes a complete set of reference documents including an Operations Manual, which provides the purpose, authorities, operational period duration, threats, and other details of significance. These guide the process of implementing the preferred method of performing a single or multiple interrelated functions in a controlled and uniform manner.

Status report: Information specifically related to the status of one or more resources, such as its availability, maintenance progress, or location.

Strategic National Stockpile (SNS): Congress appropriated funds in 1998 under the National Pharmaceutical Stockpile (NPS) program for the Centers for Disease Control to acquire a pharmaceutical and vaccine stockpile to counter CBRNE (chemical, biological, radiological, nuclear, or high-yield explosive) agents that could compromise the health of large populations of people. The name was later changed to Strategic National Stockpile (SNS) as the program expanded to include items other than pharmaceuticals. The SNS now contains antibiotics, chemical antidotes, antitoxins, life-support medications, intravenous fluids, airway maintenance supplies, and various medical and surgical items. The purpose of the SNS is to supplement and resupply state and local public health agencies in the event of a national emergency.

Strategy: A general plan or direction selected to accomplish the desired incident objectives.

Strike team: A team comprised of resources of the same kind and type that have an established minimum number of personnel, common communications, and an established leader.

Supervisor: The ICS title for an individual responsible for a division or group.

Support resources: All other resources required for support during and after an incident, such as food, tents, supplies, communications equipment, and fleet vehicles.

Supporting agency: An agency that provides resources and/or support assistance to another agency involved in the response efforts.

Supporting technology: Any form of technology that can be utilized in support of NIMS response efforts. Examples include cloud computing, infrared technologies, ortho-photo mapping, mobile computing pads, remote automatic weather stations, and various forms of cell phone communications.

System: An orderly organization and integration of any combination of resources, policies, procedures, or methods of communication to achieve a specific purpose.

Tactics: The deployment and directing of resource placement and utilization during response efforts to accomplish the objectives designated in the strategy.

Tactical resources: Personnel and major items of equipment that are available or potentially available to the operations function or for assignment to incidents. They can be classified as assigned, available, or out of service.

Task force: Operates with common communications and a designated leader in support of a specific mission or operational need. A task force may be comprised of any combination of resources required.

Technical specialist: An individual who possesses special skills and certifications which are transferable to any section of the ICS organization in need of his or her special skills.

Technology standards: Standard technology characteristics, performance parameters, conditions, or guideline specifications required to ensure compatibility, interoperability, and portability of major systems across geographic, functional, and jurisdictional lines. This often requires a review by technology support specialists.

Terrorism: According to the Homeland Security Act of 2002, terrorism is any activity that involves an act that is dangerous to human life or potentially destructive of critical infrastructure or key resources; is a violation of the criminal laws of the United States or of any State or other subdivision of the United States; and appears to be intended to intimidate or coerce a civilian population to influence the policy of a government by intimidation or coercion, or to affect the conduct of a government by mass destruction, assassination, or kidnapping.

Threat: A natural or man-made agent, individual, organization, act, or other entity that is directed at the potential to inflict harm to life, property, communications systems, operations, or the environment.

Tools: The capabilities and instruments utilized that permit the performance and completion of assigned tasks. This includes such entities as information systems, agreements, various machines, doctrinal materials, and legislative instruments.

Transfer of command: This is the procedure for command transfer from one IC to another IC. It always involves a transfer of command briefing, which may be in a written or oral format.

Tribal: Any Native American Indian nation, band, tribe, or other organized group or community recognized as eligible for the special programs and services provided by the United States government.

Type: An Incident Command System resource classification that refers to capability. Generally—on a scale numbered from type 1 to type 4—type 1 is the most capable and type 4 the least capable of the resources. This designation of type 1, 2, 3, or 4 is based upon a resource's size, power, capacity, or the qualifications and experience of personnel.

Unified approach: The integration and coordination of command, resource, communications, and information management components into a functional and effective systematic approach to response activities.

Unified area command: This command structure is formed when the incidents under an area command are or become multijurisdictional.

Unified command: The responding agencies and jurisdictions with responsibility for the incident and share the incident management command. The more senior members of the involved agencies work to establish a common set of objectives and strategies and a single Incident Action Plan (IAP).

Unit: The organization element that has functional responsibility for a designated and specific incident planning, logistics, or finance/administration activity.

Unit leader: The ICS functional section individual charged with managing a specific functional sectional unit.

Unity of command: Every individual is accountable to only one designated supervisor to whom they report at the scene of an incident. The chain of command and unity of command clarifies the reporting relationships and eliminates the confusion created by multiple, conflicting directives. It applies to orders but does not apply to information exchange and sharing. Incident command managers must be able to control all subordinates under their span of control.

Vital records: These maintained records are essential for meeting operational needs during disasters, emergencies, or incident conditions. They are used to preserve fiscal and legal rights of individual citizens and governmental entities.

Volunteer: With respect to the NIMS, this is any individual who has volunteered and been accepted by the lead agency to perform services without the promise, expectation, or receipt of any form of compensation for the services performed.

Figures

Commonly Used Acronyms

ACF	Administration for Children and Families
AHRQ	Agency for Healthcare Research and Quality
ALS	Advanced Life Support
AoA	Administration on Aging
ATSDR	Agency for Toxic Substances and Disease Registry
CBRNE	Chemical, Biological, Radiological, Nuclear, or High-Yield Explosive
CDC	Centers for Disease Control and Prevention
CMS	Centers for Medicare and Medicaid Services
COOP	Continuity of Operations Plan
COP	Common Operating Picture
DEA	Drug Enforcement Agency
DHHS	Department of Health and Human Services
DHS	Department of Homeland Security
DMORT	Disaster Mortuary Operational Response Team
DOC	Department Operations Center
DOD	Department of Defense
DSCA	Defense Support to Civil Authority
EMAC	Emergency Management Assistance Compact
EOC	Emergency Operations Center
EOP	Emergency Operations Plan
EPI	Emergency Public Information
EPLOS	Emergency Preparedness Liaison Officers
FDA	Food and Drug Administration
FEMA	Federal Emergency Management Agency
FOG	Field Operations Guide
FORSCOM	United States Army Forces Command
FY	Fiscal Year
GIS	Global Information System
HAZMAT	Hazardous Material
HICS	Hospital Incident Command System

HPP	Hospital Preparedness Program
HRSA	Health Resources and Services Administration
HSPD-5	Homeland Security Presidential Directive – 5
HSPD-8	Homeland Security Presidential Directive – 8
IAP	Incident Action Plan
IC	Incident Commander
ICP	Incident Command Post
ICS	Incident Command System
IC	Incident Command
IMT	Incident Management Team
IOM	Institute of Medicine
IHS	Indian Health Service
IMT	Incident Management Team
JFCOM	Joint Forces Command
JFO	Joint Field Office
JIC	Joint Information Center
JIS	Joint Information System
JTF	Joint Task Force
LNO	Liaison Officer
MAC	Multi-Agency Coordination
MACS	Multi-Agency Coordination System
MRE	Meals Ready to Eat
NDMS	National Disaster Medical System
NGO	Nongovernmental organization
NIC	National Integration Center
NIH	National Institutes of Health
NIMS	National Incident Management System
NRP	National Response Plan
NRP-CIA	Catastrophic Incident Annex to the National Response Plan
NRP-CIS	Catastrophic Incident Supplement to the National Response Plan
OSD	Office of the Secretary of Defense
OSHA	Occupational Safety and Health Administration
PAO	Public Affairs Officer
POLREP	Pollution Report
PIO	Public Information Officer
PVO	Private Voluntary Organizations

R&D	Research and development
RESTAT	Resources Status
ROE	Rules of Engagement
ROSS	Resource Ordering and Status System
SAMHSA	Substance Abuse and Mental Health Services Administration
SDO	Standards Development Organizations
SEOC	State Emergency Operations Center
SHIP	State Health Improvement Plan
SITREP	Situation Report
SO	Safety Officer
SOG	Standard Operating Guidelines
SOP	Standard Operating Procedure
TA	Technical Assistance
UAC	Unified Area Command
UASI	Urban Area Security Initiative
UC	Unified Command
US&R	Urban Search and Rescue

Resources

Websites of Interest

Agency for Toxic Substances and Disease Registry www.atsdr.cdc.gov
American Red Cross www.redcross.org
Association of State and Territorial Health Officials www.astho.org
Centers for Disease Control and Prevention www.cdc.gov
Citizen Corps www.citizencorps.gov
Department of Energy www.energy.gov
Department of Health and Human Services www.hhs.gov/disasters
Department of Homeland Security www.dhs.gov
Department of Justice www.justice.gov
Environmental Protection Agency www.epa.gov
Federal Emergency Management Agency www.fema.gov
Food and Drug Administration www.fda.gov
Institute for Business and Home Safety www.ibhs.org
National Fire Protection Agency www.nfpa.org
National Mass Fatalities Institute www.nmfi.org
National Oceanographic and Atmospheric Administration www.noaa.gov
National Safety Compliance www.osha-safety-training.net
National Weather Service www.nws.noaa.gov
Naval Postgraduate School www.nps.org
Nuclear Regulatory Commission www.nrc.gov
The Critical Infrastructure Assurance Office www.ciao.gov
The White House www.whitehouse.gov/response
United States Department of Agriculture www.usda.gov
United States Fire Administration www.usfa.fema.gov

Bibliography

Books of Interest

Beckstrom, Rod, and Ori Brafman. *The Starfish and the Spider.* New York: Penguin, 2006.

Flynn, Stephen. The Edge of Disaster. Random House, 2007.

Honore, Lt. Gen. Russel. *Survival.* Atria Books, 2009.

Jerome, Fred, and Rodger Taylor. *Einstein on Race and Racism.* Rutgers University Press, 2005.

Koenig, Harold G. *In the Wake of Disaster.* Templeton Foundation Press, 2006.

Kubler-Ross, Elizabeth. *On Death and Dying.* Routledge, 1969.

Lewis, Ted. *Critical Infrastructure Protection in Homeland Security.* John Wiley & Sons, 2006.

Norwitz, Jeffrey, ed. *Armed Groups: Studies in National Security, Counterterrorism, and Counterinsurgency.* Naval War College Press, 2008.

Taleb, Nassim Nicholas. *The Black Swan.* Random House, 2007.

Federal Documents and Journal Articles of Interest

Arnold, Damon T. 'The Need for Public Health Fusion Centers.' *Journal of Homeland Security,* November 2007.

Agency for Healthcare Research and Quality: 'Recommendations for a national mass patient and evacuee movement, regulating, and tracking

225

system.' AHQR Publication No. AHQR-09-0039-EF, 2009a. Rockville, MD: AHQR.

Bell, Carl C. 'Social and Emotional Costs of Learning Disabilities—Perspective.' 165, no. 2 (2008):

174-75.

Gould, Stephen Jay, and Niles Eldredge. 'Punctuated Equilibria: The tempo and mode of evolution reconsidered.' *Paleobiology* 3 (1972), 115-51.

IOM (Institute of Medicine). *Emergency medical services: At the crossroads.* Washington, DC: The National Academies Press. Accessed October 8, 2010. http://www.nap.edu/catalog.php?record_id=11629.

IOM Forum on Medical and Public Health Preparedness for Catastrophic Events: 'Medical Surge Capacity.' Workshop Summary Institute of Medicine of the National Academy of Sciences Press, 2010

IOM Forum on Medical and Public Health Preparedness for Catastrophic Events: 'The Public Health Emergency Medical Countermeasures Enterprise: Innovative Strategies to Enhance Products from Discovery through Approval;' Workshop Summary Institute of Medicine of the National Academy of Sciences Press, 2010.

IOM Forum on Medical Countermeasures Dispensing: National Academy of Sciences Press, 2010.

IOM Workshop Series: 'The 2009 H1N1 Influenza Vaccination Campaign.' National Academy of Sciences Press, 2010.

IOM Workshop Series: 'Crisis Standards of Care.' National Academy of Sciences Press, 2010.

Appendix A. Emergency Response Kit Components

Use the checklist below for community intervention and disaster and emergency response work.

Basic Tools

Flashlight
Portable radio
GPS guidance device

Food and Water

- Store at least a two-week supply of food and water.
- In the disaster environment, one's need for both water and calories may greatly increase.
- High-calorie, nutritious foods are desirable as they offer more calories and are easier to carry.
- Select foods requiring *no* refrigeration, preparation, or cooking.
- Check for individual allergies with any foods selected and appropriately avoid their use.
- *Avoid* containers that decompose, glass (breaks), and heavy metal containers (must be carried).
- One (1) gallon of water per person per day.
- Two (2) quarts for drinking water; 2 quarts for food preparation and sanitation.
- Nonperishable pasteurized milk (2% cow's, soy, etc.).
- Nondegradable packets of various juices.
- Water-filtering devices and replacement filters.
- Manual can opener and disposable eating utensils.
- Ready-to-eat packaged meats, fruits, and vegetables.
- Protein, granola, and fruit bars; unsalted nuts and dried fruits.

- Dry cereal.
- Peanut butter.
- Unsalted crackers.
- Foods for those with special nutritional needs.
- Baby foods (if required).
- Vitamins; dietary enzymes if desired.
- Pet foods.

Medical Records, Supplies, and Equipment

- Individual and family emergency health records. Each individual should be identified by full name, date of birth, blood type, and other required medical insurance information. Indicate any allergies, past or current medical problems, surgeries, and prescription medication requirements.
- The medication information should include current dosages and timing of medication administration. All recommended vaccinations should be kept up-to-date and the date of administration recorded. Any individual special needs should be noted.
- Soap and alcohol-based sanitation products (such as wipes and gels).
- Prescribed medical equipment (such as blood sugar and blood pressure monitoring devices).
- Latex-free sterile gloves.
- Nonbreakable thermometer.
- Be sure to read and follow all medication information and prescribing sheets provided.
- All prescribed medications (keep a two-month supply).
- Medications for fever (such as acetaminophen or aspirin). Please note: Ibuprofen does not reduce fever.
- Antacid and antidiarrheal medications.
- Fluids with electrolytes.
- Plastic garbage bags for sanitation.
- Tissues, toilet paper, and disposable diapers.

Appendix B. Terms Utilized in Complementary and Alternative Medicine

Listed below are common terms utilized in complementary and alternative medicine.

Acupressure: A form of massage in which acupuncture points are stimulated without the use of inserting acupuncture needles.

Acupuncture: A science that involves the manipulation and optimization of healthy Qi flow through a network of bodily channels by the insertion of needles at specific acupuncture points.

Allopathic medicine: This involves the use of traditional Western medical practices.

Antioxidants: Chemical substances that act block or minimize the effects of free radical chemicals produced within the body.

Aromatherapy: The use of specific scents of natural origin to improve the health and well-being of individuals facing potential threats to their health.

Asana: This involves assuming postures that support the practice of meditation to improve overall health of the practitioner.

Atherosclerosis: The pathological buildup of plaque within blood vessels, such as arteries, that impedes the flow of blood.

Ayurveda: A medical practice that involves the balancing of the various fluids and substances within the body to achieve optimal health.

Biofeedback: An interactive program, often computer guided, utilized to train individuals to relax and thereby improve their health by lowering their heart rate, blood pressure, and breathing rate.

Bodywork: Any of various forms of practice directed at working with an individual's physical make-up to improve his or her health.

Chiropractic: The manipulation of the skeletal structures, joints, and muscles to improve an individual's health.

Complementary medicine: The blending of Western and Eastern medical concepts to optimize their positive benefits.

Diabetes: A disease state in which the body does not produce enough of the hormone insulin, which is required to maintain normal blood and tissues sugar levels.

Environmental toxins: Any chemical agent within the environment capable of producing harm.

Enzymes: Protein-based substances that catalyze chemical reactions within the body.

Essential fatty acids: These are fatty acids that the body does not normally produce and are required within the diet to maintain an individual's health.

Essential oils: Oils that are believed to be essential by some practitioners in order for the body to maintain its health.

Feng shui: The Chinese concept of the creation, designing, and placement of structures that allow for the flow and balancing of energy in the home and surrounding environment.

Fluoridation: The use of fluorine gas, which is dissolved in water, to enhance dental resistance to the development of cavities.

Free radicals: Harmful chemicals that result from metabolic processes that are ultimately toxic to the body.

Ginseng: An herb used for its medicinal properties in various forms.

Hatha yoga: The branch of yoga that deals with the body via various postures, breathing exercises, and other techniques.

Heart failure: When the heart is unable to pump blood out in a sufficient quantity to meet basic bodily needs.

Heavy metals: Various metallic elements that are harmful to the body when contact with a sufficient amount occurs.

Herbal medicine: The use of various herbal medicinal plants to prevent and treat various injuries, ailments, and diseases.

High blood pressure: The result of too much pressure being exerted by the heart as it circulates blood through the body and is affected by the heart rate as well.

High-density lipoproteins (HDLs): These are the 'healthy' lipid-protein complexes in the blood that act to remove harmful fatty substance wastes, which can deposit in bodily tissues and clog blood vessels.

Homeostasis: The regulated balancing, normalization, and maintenance of bodily chemistry and structural and functional systems.

Hormones: A substance produced by a group of cells that exerts effects on distant target sites within the body.

Hypertension: When too much tension is produced by the heart muscles as they strain to circulate blood and can result in high blood pressure. See 'high blood pressure' above.

Hyperthermia: When the body temperature exceeds the upper limits of normal, which can sometimes be life threatening.

Low-density lipoproteins (LDLs): Lipid-protein complexes obtained from food sources, which contain harmful substances that result in the production of waste products that can deposit in bodily tissues and clog blood vessels.

Mantra: A series of words or sounds that assist in the process of meditation and self-realization.

Massage: Hands-on manipulations of a recipient's body by a practitioner who has been trained in various techniques and methods of a healing art discipline.

Meridians: Vessels that have been noted in Chinese medical practice to transport Chi (energy) throughout the body.

Mineral: Trace elements that are essential for supporting normal health and are normally obtained in food sources.

Nutritional supplement: Products that contain nutritional sources intended to supplement a person's usual dietary practices.

Osteopathy: Related to injury, illness, or disease that involves the bones of the body.

Placebo effect: Occurs when a substance causes a response in a positive or negative direction based on a person's belief that it will.

Protein: A chemical substance within the body made up of a series of amino acids.

Qi (Ki): Pronounced 'key,' this is the 'life energy' recognized within the realm of Chinese medicine as underlying all life forms. Also represents air, as in a breath.

Qigong: Translated as 'energy exercise' or 'breath work.' There are thousands of exercises of this type noted in Chinese medicine.

Reflexology: The use of massage techniques upon various parts of a person's body to improve health.

Shiatsu: The application of pressure utilizing finger or solid objects to impart a positive healing effect through manipulation of acupressure points, which closely align with acupuncture points.

Stress: The accumulation of emotional discomfort arising from a physical or psychic origin.

Tai Chi: A series of coordinated movements that comprise a flowing form of Qigong.

Transcendental meditation (TM): A form of meditation that transcends the physical realities of the world to reach a deepened understanding of existence as a sentient being.

Trigger-point massage: Pressure applied to skin utilizing various message techniques to increase blood flow in muscles and other bodily structures.

Ultraviolet (UV) light: A high-energy light that is part of sunlight and is essential for life forms to exist but can be harmful with overexposure.

Vitamin: A group of chemical agents that serve as substrates for various metabolic cycles within the body and are essential for life and health.

Yin and yang: Two opposing forces that are both essential and must be in proper balance to support life.

Yoga: A series of movements and postures performed to balance and maintain a practitioner's health and well-being.

Zen: The oriental art of fully living in the moment without attachments to the past or future.

Appendix C. The Bill of Rights

FIRST AMENDMENT: Congress shall make no law respecting an establishment of religion, or prohibiting the free exercise thereof, or abridging the freedom of speech, or of the press; or the right of the people peaceably to assemble, and to petition the Government for a redress of grievances.

SECOND AMENDMENT: A well regulated Militia, being necessary to the security of a free State, the right of the people to keep and bear Arms, shall not be infringed.

THIRD AMENDMENT: No Soldier shall, in time of peace be quartered in any house, without the consent of the Owner, nor in time of war, but in a manner to be prescribed by law.

FOURTH AMENDMENT: The right of the people to be secure in their persons, houses, papers, and effects, against unreasonable searches and seizures, shall not be violated, and no Warrants shall issue, but upon probable cause, supported by Oath of affirmation, and particularly describing the place to be searched, and the persons or things to be seized.

FIFTH AMENDMENT: No person shall be held to answer for a capitol, or otherwise infamous crime, unless on a presentment or indictment of a Grand Jury, except in cases arising in the land or naval forces, or in the Militia, when in actual service in time of War or public danger; nor shall any person be subject for the same offense to be twice put in jeopardy of life or limb; nor shall be compelled in any criminal case to be a witness against himself, nor be deprived of life, liberty, or property, without due process of law; nor shall private property be taken for public use, without just compensation.

SIXTH AMENDMENT: In all criminal prosecutions, the accused shall enjoy the right to a speedy and public trial, by an impartial jury of the State and district wherein the crime shall have been committed, which district shall have been previously ascertained by law, and to be informed of the nature and cause of the accusation; to be confronted with the witnesses against him; to have compulsory process for obtaining witnesses in his favor, and to have the Assistance of Counsel for his defense.

SEVENTH AMENDMENT: In suits at common law, where the value in controversy shall exceed twenty dollars, the right of trial by jury shall be preserved, and no fact tried by a jury, shall be otherwise re-examined in any Court of the United States, than according to the rules of the common law.

EIGHTH AMENDMENT: Excessive bail shall not be required, nor excessive fines imposed, nor cruel and unusual punishments inflicted.

NINTH AMENDMENT: The enumeration in the Constitution, of certain rights, shall not be construed to deny or disparage others retained by the people.

TENTH AMENDMENT: The powers not delegated to the United States by the Constitution, nor prohibited by it to the States, are reserved to the States respectively, or to the people.

NOTES PAGE

NOTES PAGE

NOTES PAGE

NOTES PAGE

About the Author

Col. Damon T. Arnold, MD, MPH, CMT (Ret.) was appointed as the 16th director of the Illinois Department of Public Health on October 1, 2007, where he operated an agency of over 1,100 employees with an annual budget of over 600 million dollars. The agency was responsible for the public health concerns of the approximately 12.5 million residents within, and millions of annual travelers to, the state of Illinois. During his four years in this position, he brought millions of dollars to the state of Illinois and was very active on the local, state, and federal levels.

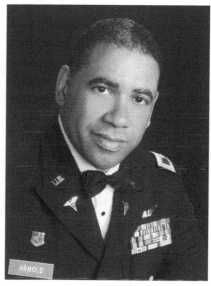

Dr. Arnold obtained his undergraduate degree from Howard University in Washington, DC, and both his MD and MPH degrees from the University of Illinois in Chicago. He completed his residency in internal medicine at Cook County Hospital, followed by a residency in occupational medicine. He served as the Medical Director for over 25 years in private hospital and health care systems in Chicago. Dr. Arnold also served for 26 years in the Army National Guard, where he served as the commander of the Joint Medical Command Task Force and State Surgeon General for over 12 years. He completed 17 overseas missions that included locations in Africa, Central America, South America, Europe, the Middle East, and Asia.

He was awarded the highly coveted Military Legion of Merit Medal by President Barack Obama for his military achievements. Dr. Arnold also was awarded three Army Commendation Medals for his wartime deployments to Iraq and Kuwait, where he served as the officer in charge of battlefield medical operations. During these deployments, he functioned as a mechanized infantry combat medic as well as a qualified flight surgeon on over 120 field and flight operations. Among numerous medals, he also received two National Defense Service Medals as well as awards on the battlefield. He has completed formal training in holistic medicine for therapeutic massage therapy and acupuncture. He has received over 60 major awards in the fields of public health and medicine.

Dr. Arnold served as a member of several health care focus groups, including the Harvard University LAMPS Committee, Institute of Medicine in Washington, DC, Association of State and Territorial Health Officials, and several federally based organizations. He has published many articles and contributed to books over the years. He is currently serving as the associate dean for the College of Health Sciences and the director of the public health graduate program at Chicago State University. He is also an adjunct professor at the University of Illinois, College of Medicine, and the School of Public Health. He lives with his wife, Sharon Johnson-Arnold, in Chicago and has several hobbies, including writing and art.